Human Reproduction at a Glance

Human Reproduction at a Glance

LINDA J. HEFFNER

MD, PhD

Associate Professor of Obstetrics, Gynecology and
    Reproductive Biology at Harvard Medical School
Director of Maternal–Fetal Medicine
Department of Obstetrics and Gynecology
Brigham & Women's Hospital
Boston
USA

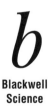

Blackwell
Science

© 2001 by
Blackwell Science Ltd
Editorial Offices:
Osney Mead, Oxford OX2 0EL
25 John Street, London WC1N 2BS
23 Ainslie Place, Edinburgh EH3 6AJ
350 Main Street, Malden
  MA 02148-5018, USA
54 University Street, Carlton
  Victoria 3053, Australia
10, rue Casimir Delavigne
  75006 Paris, France

Other Editorial Offices:
Blackwell Wissenschafts-Verlag GmbH
Kurfürstendamm 57
10707 Berlin, Germany

Blackwell Science KK
MG Kodenmacho Building
7–10 Kodenmacho Nihombashi
Chuo-ku, Tokyo 104, Japan

Iowa State University Press
A Blackwell Science Company
2121 S. State Avenue
Ames, Iowa 50014-8300, USA

First published 2001

Set by Graphicraft Limited, Hong Kong
Printed and bound in Great Britain
by MPG Books Ltd, Bodmin, Cornwall

The Blackwell Science logo is a
trade mark of Blackwell Science Ltd,
registered at the United Kingdom
Trade Marks Registry

DISTRIBUTORS

Marston Book Services Ltd
PO Box 269
Abingdon, Oxon OX14 4YN
(*Orders*: Tel: 01235 465500
      Fax: 01235 465555)

USA
Blackwell Science, Inc.
Commerce Place
350 Main Street
Malden, MA 02148-5018
(*Orders*: Tel: 800 759 6102
      781 388 8250
      Fax: 781 388 8255)

Canada
Login Brothers Book Company
324 Saulteaux Crescent
Winnipeg, Manitoba R3J 3T2
(*Orders*: Tel: 204 837 2987)

Australia
Blackwell Science Pty Ltd
54 University Street
Carlton, Victoria 3053
(*Orders*: Tel: 3 9347 0300
      Fax: 3 9347 5001)

A catalogue record for this title
is available from the British Library

ISBN 0-632-05461-1

Library of Congress
Cataloging-in-Publication Data
Heffner, Linda.
  Human reproduction at a glance / Linda J. Heffner.
    p.; cm.
  Includes index.
  ISBN 0-632-05461-1
    1. Human reproduction. 2. Reproductive health. I. Title.
    [DNLM: 1. Reproduction—physiology. 2. Genital Diseases, Female.
  3. Pregnancy Complications. 4. Sexually Transmitted Diseases.
  WQ 205 H461h 2001]
  QP251 .H39 2001
  612.6—dc21   00-054372

For further information on
Blackwell Science, visit our website:
www.blackwell-science.com

Contents

Preface

Having taught reproductive medicine to medical students for over 20 years, I found the necessary information on the human reproductive processes and their diseases to be scattered over textbooks of anatomy, embryology and development, obstetrics and gynecology and surgery. *Human Reproduction at a Glance* was written as a learning and study guide for medical students and physicians who wish to have a comprehensive, but easy to use, overview of the anatomy, physiology and pathophysiology of the reproductive processes in both sexes.

For ease of use, the book is divided into two parts. Part I, which consists of 22 chapters, covers normal human reproduction beginning with the embryology of the reproductive tracts, through puberty with the resulting mature male and female anatomy and physiology, through fertilization, pregnancy and menopause. Part II, which consists of 20 chapters, covers the pathophysiology of anatomic, physiologic and psychologic disorders interfering with normal reproductive function or health. Six chapters are devoted to the more common malignancies involving the reproductive organs.

Like other books in the series, *Human Reproduction at a Glance* is written so that each topic is confined to a discrete vignette with appropriate illustrations or tables in a single or facing page format. In Part II, each topic also follows a standard format of description of the disorder, its epidemiology, pathophysiology and, whenever it aids in understanding the disorder, a brief description of the commonly used treatments.

Assembling a book of this breadth is a major undertaking and many people contributed to this process. I would like to thank the students in the Harvard Medical School Class of 2002 for their many helpful comments. Additionally, I would like to thank the following individuals at Harvard Medical School without whose help this book never would have been written: my husband, Dr Douglas Richardson, who served both as a clinical resource and as a personal editor; Dr Ross Berkowitz for his comments on gestational trophoblastic disease and endometrial cancer; Dr Daniel Federman, for reading and commenting on the entirety of Part I when I only asked him to look it over; Dr Marc Garnick, for his comments on prostate diseases; Dr Daniel George, for his helpful comments on testicular cancer, Dr Carolyn Kaelin, for her input into the breast cancer section; Dr Michael Muto, for editing the ovarian cancer section; Dr Ellen Sheets, for her input into the section on cervical cancer and finally, Dr Ari van Tienhoven, my teacher and mentor from my beginning days of teaching reproductive physiology at Cornell University.

Books never appear in print without publishers and I would like to thank Bridgette Jones, Meg Barton, Fiona Goodgame and Dr Michael Stein at Blackwell Science for their encouragement and professionalism in bringing the project to fruition. Special thanks are sent to the illustrator, Mike Elms, who did a marvelous job of converting a hodge-podge of illustrations into a cohesive series.

Linda J. Heffner
Boston, 2001

Table and Figure Acknowledgements

The darkfield images of egg and sperm on the cover were kindly provided by Dr Catherine Racowsky, Director of the Assisted Reproduction Laboratory at Brigham and Women's Hospital.

The following tables and figures have been redrawn from the originals and were used with permission of the publishers. Every effort has been made by the author and the publishers to contact all the copyright holders to obtain their permission to reproduce copyright material. However, if any have been inadvertently overlooked, the publisher will be pleased to make the necessary arrangements at the first opportunity.

2 Gonadotropins

Figure 2.1: Braunstein, G. (1989) Placental hormones, hormonal preparation for and control of parturition, and hormonal diagnosis of pregnancy. In: *Endocrinology* (ed. L.J. deGroot), p. 2045. W.B. Saunders & Co., Philadelphia.

Figure 2.2: Halvorsen, L.M., Chin, W.W. (1999) Gonadotropic hormones: biosynthesis, secretion, receptors, and action. In: *Reproductive Endocrinology* (eds S.S.C. Yen, R.B. Jaffe, R.L. Barbieri), p 92. W.B. Saunders & Co., Philadelphia.

3 Steroid and hormone biosynthesis

Figure 3.1: Dr Susan Haas, Harvard Vanguard Health Plan and Brigham and Women's Hospital, Boston.

Figure 3.2: Yeh, J., Adashi, E.Y. (1999) The ovarian life cycle. In: *Reproductive Endocrinology* (eds S.S.C. Yen, R.B. Jaffe, R.L. Barbieri), p. 168. W.B. Saunders & Co., Philadelphia.

4 Steroid hormone mechanism of action and metabolism

Figure 4.1: O'Malley, B.W., Strott, C.A. (1999) Steroid hormones: metabolism and mechanism of action. In: *Reproductive Endocrinology* (eds S.S.C. Yen, R.B. Jaffe, R.L. Barbieri), p. 124. W.B. Saunders & Co., Philadelphia.

5 Embryology of the reproductive tract

Figure 5.1: Johnson, M.H., Everitt, B.J. (1995) *Essential Reproduction*, p. 4. Blackwell Science, Oxford and

Morton, C.C., Miron, P. (1999) Cytogenetics. In: *Reproduction in Reproductive Endocrinology* (eds S.S.C. Yen, R.B. Jaffe, R.L. Barbieri), p. 337. W.B. Saunders & Co., Philadelphia.

Figure 5.2: Williams, P.L., Wendell-Smith, C.P., Treadgold, S. (1966) *Basic Human Embryology*, p. 76. J.B. Lippincott & Co., Philadelphia.

Figure 5.3: Balinsky, B.I. (1970) *An Introduction to Embryology*, 3rd edn, p. 497. W.B. Saunders & Co., Philadelphia.

Figure 5.4: Williams, P.L., Wendell-Smith, C.P., Treadgold, S. (1996) *Basic Human Embryology*, p. 78. J.B. Lippincott & Co. Philadelphia.

6 Gross anatomy of the male reproductive tract

Figure 6.1: Romanes, G.J. (1972) *Cunningham's Textbook of Anatomy*, 11th edn, pp. 525, 531, 533. Oxford University Press, Oxford.

7 Microscopic anatomy of the male reproductive tract

Figure 7.1: Bloom, W., Fawcett, D.W. (1969) *A Textbook of Histology*, 9th edn, p. 688. W.B. Saunders & Co., Philadelphia.

Figure 7.2: Clermont, Y. (1972) Kinetics of spermatogenesis in mammals: seminiferous epithelium cycle and spermatogonial renewal. *Physiol Rev* **52** : 206.

Figure 7.3: Johnson, M.H., Everitt, B.J. (1995) *Essential Reproduction*, p. 53. Blackwell Science, Oxford.

8 Gross anatomy of the female reproductive tract

Figure 8.1: Netter, F.H. (1954) *The Ciba Collection of Medical Illustrations*: *Vol. 2, The Reproductive System*, p. 110.

Figure 8.2: Romanes, G.J. (1972) *Cunningham's Textbook of Anatomy*, 11th edn, p. 544. Oxford University Press, Oxford.

9 Microscopic anatomy of the female reproductive tract

Figure 9.1: Turner, C.D. (1966) *General Endocrinology*, 5th edn, p. 400. W.B. Saunders & Co., Philadelphia.

Figure 9.2: Netter, F.H. (1954) *The Ciba Collection of Medical Illustrations: Volume 2, The Reproductive System*, pp. 115, 118–19.

10 Puberty in boys

Figures 10.1 and 10.2: Marshall, W.A., Tanner, J.M. (1970) Variations in pattern of pubertal changes in boys. *Arch Dis Child* **45** : 13–23.

11 Puberty in girls

Figures 11.1 and 11.2: Marshall, W.A., Tanner, J.M. (1969) Variations in pattern of pubertal changes in girls. *Arch Dis Child* **44** : 291–301.

12 Male reproductive physiology

Figure 12.1: Jordan, G.H. (1999) Erectile function and dysfunction. *Postgrad Med* **105** : 133.

Figure 12.2: Guiliano, F.A., Rampin, O., Benoit, G., Jardin, A. (1995) Neural control of penile erection. *Urol Clin North Am* **22** : 748.

13 The menstrual cycle

Figure 13.1: Groome, N.P., Illingworth, P.J., O'Brien, M. *et al.* (1996) Measurement of dimeric inhibin B throughout the human menstrual cycle. *J Clin Endocrinol Metab* **81** : 1401–1405 and

Marshall, J.C., Odell, W.D. (1989) The menstrual cycle—hormonal regulation, mechanisms of anovulation and responses of the reproductive tract to steroid hormones. In: *Endocrinology* (ed. L. DeGroot), p. 1946. W.B. Saunders & Co., Philadelphia.

14 Human sexual response

Figure 14.1: Masters, W.H., Johnson, V.E. (1966) *Human Sexual Response*, p. 5. Little, Brown & Co., Boston.

15 Reproductive genetics

Figure 15.1: Johnson, M.H., Everitt, B.J. (1995) *Essential Reproduction*, p. 2. Blackwell Science, Oxford.

16 Fertilization and establishment of pregnancy

Figure 16.1: Alberts, B., Bray, D., Lewis, J. *et al.* (1994) *Molecular Biology of the Cell*, p. 1031. Garland Publishing, New York.

17 Endocrinology of pregnancy

Figure 17.1: Yen, S.S.C. (1989) Endocrinology of pregnancy. In: *Maternal–Fetal Medicine*, (eds R.K. Creasy, R. Resnik), 2nd edn, p. 385. W.B. Saunders & Co., Philadelphia.

Figure 17.2: Jaffe, R.B. (1999) Neuroendocrine-metabolic regulation of pregnancy. In: *Reproductive Endocrinology* (eds S.S.C. Yen, R.B. Jaffe, R.L. Barbieri), p. 767. W.B. Saunders & Co., Philadelphia.

Figure 17.3: Liu, J.H., Rebar, R.W. (1999) Endocrinology of pregnancy. In: *Maternal–Fetal Medicine*, 4th edn (eds R.K. Creasy, R. Resnik), p. 386. W.B. Saunders & Co., Philadelphia.

Figures 17.4, 17.5, 17.6: Yen, S.S.C. (1989) Endocrinology of pregnancy. In: *Maternal–Fetal Medicine*, 2nd edn (R.K. Creasy, R. Resnik), pp. 377, 380, 382. W.B. Saunders & Co., Philadelphia.

19 Labor

Figure 19.1: Norwitz, E.R., Robinson, J.N., Challis, J.G.R. (1999) The control of labor. *N Engl J Med* **341** : 662.

Figure 19.2: Challis, J.R.G., Gibb, W. (1996) Control of parturition. *Prenat Neonat Med* **1** : 284.

20 The breast and lactation

Figure 20.1: Lyons, W.P. (1958) Hormonal synergism in mammary growth. *Proc R Soc Lond B* **149** : 303.

Figure 20.2: Worthington-Roberts, B.S. (1997) Lactation: basic considerations. In: *Nutrition in Pregnancy and Lactation* (eds B.S. Worthington-Roberts, S.R. Williams), 6th edn, p. 320. Brown & Benchmark Publishers, Madison.

24 Abnormalities of male sexual differentiation and development

Figure 24.1: Williams, P.L., Wendell-Smith, C.P., Treadgold, S. (1966) *Basic Human Embryology*, p. 81. J.B. Lippincott & Co., Philadelphia.

Table 24.1: Griffin, J.E. (1992) Androgen resistance—the clinical and molecular spectrum. *N Eng J Med* **326** : 612.

25 Abnormalities of femal sexual differentiation and development

Figure 25.1: Williams, P.L., Wendell-Smith, C.P., Treadgold, S. (1966) *Basic Human Embryology*, p. 81. J.B. Lippincott & Co., Philadelphia.

26 Precocious puberty

Tables 26.1 and 26.2: Miller, W.L., Styne, D.M. (1999) Female puberty and its disorders. In: *Reproductive Endocrinology* (eds S.C.C. Yen, R.B. Jaffe, R.L. Barbieri), pp. 394, 397. W.B. Saunders & Co., Philadelphia.

27 Delayed or absent puberty

Table 27.1: Miller, W.L., Styne, D.M. (1999) Female puberty and its disorders. In: *Reproductive Endocrinology* (eds Yen, S.C.C., R.B. Jaffe, R.L. Barbieri), p. 401. W.B. Saunders & Co., Philadelphia.

28 Amenorrhea

Figures 28.1 and 28.2: Barbieri, R.L. (1997) Approach to menstrual disorders and galactorrhea. In: *Textbook of Internal Medicine* (ed. W.N. Kelley), 3rd edn, pp. 2146–47. Lippincott-Raven Publishers, Philadelphia.

29 Hirsutism and androgenetic alopecia

Figures 29.1 and 29.2: Yen, S.S.C. (1999) Polycystic ovary syndrome. In: *Reproductive Endocrinology* (eds S.C.C. Yen, R.B. Jaffe, R.L. Barbieri), p. 458. W.B. Saunders & Co., Philadelphia.

30 Hyperprolactinemia

Figure 30.1: Yen, S.S.C., Jaffe, R.B. (1999) Prolactin in human reproduction. In: *Reproductive Endocrinology* (eds S.C.C. Yen, R.B. Jaffe, R.L. Barbieri), p. 261. W.B. Saunders & Co., Philadelphia.

31 Sexual dysfunction

Figure 31.1: Kaplan, H.S. (1995) *The Sexual Desire Disorders*, p. 17. Brunner/Mazel, Publishers, New York.

33 Multifetal pregnancy

Figure 33.1: FitzGerald, M.J.T., FitzGerald, M. (1994) *Human Embryology*, p. 51. Baillière Tindall, London.

34 Pregnancy complications

Figure 34.1: Stein, Z., Kline, J., Susser, E. *et al.* (1980) Maternal age and spontaneous abortion. In: *Embryonic and Fetal Death* (eds I.H. Porter, E.B. Hook). Academic Press, New York.

Figure 34.2: Huszar, G. (1989) Physiology of the myometrium. In: *Maternal–Fetal Medicine*, 2nd edn, (eds R. Creasy, R. Resnik), p. 147. W.B. Saunders & Co., Philadelphia.

Figure 34.3: Szulman, A.E., Surti, U. (1984) The syndromes of partial and complete molar gestation. *Clin Obstet Gynecol* **27** : 177.

Table 34.1: Thompson, M.W. (1986) *Thompson and Thompson's Genetics in Medicine*, 4th edn. W.B. Saunders & Co., Philadelphia.

35 Overview of neoplasia

Figure 35.1: Thompson, T.C., Timme, T.L., Sehgal, I. (1997) The role of p53 in prostate cancer progression in accomplishments. In: *Cancer Research 1996* (eds J.G. Fortner, P.A. Sharp). Lipincott-Raven, Philadelphia.

36 Breast cancer

Tables 36.1 and 36.2: Marchant, D.J. (1997) *Risk Factors in Breast Disease* (ed. D.J. Marchant), pp. 116, 119. W.B. Saunders & Co., Philadelphia.

Figure 36.1: Lopez-Otin, C., Diamondis, E.P. (1998) Breast and prostate cancer: an analysis of common epidemiological, genetic, and biochemical features. *Endocr Rev* **19** : 383.

37 Testicular tumors

Figure 37.1: Walt, H. *et al.* (1992) Characterization of precancerous and neoplastic human testicular germ cells. In: *Pathobiology of Human Germ Cell Neoplasia,* (eds J.W. Osterhuis, Walt H., Damjanov, eds) *Rec Results Can Res* **123** : 41.

38 Disease of the prostate

Figure 38.1: Kirby, R., Christmas, T. (1993) *Anatomy, embryology and histopathology in Benign Prostatic Hypertrophy*, p. 18. Gower Medical Publishing, New York.

Figure 38.2: Lepor, H., Lawson, R.K. (1993) *Prostate Diseases*, p. 45. W.B. Saunders & Co., Philadelphia.

39 Ovarian neoplasms

Table 39.1: DiSaia, P.J., Creasman, R.K. (1997) Epithelial ovarian cancer. In: *Clinical Gynecologic Oncology*, 5th edn, p. 283. Mosby, St. Louis.

40 Endometrial cancer

Table 40.1: Mencaglia, L., Tonellotto, D., Tiso, E. (1999) Epidemiology of endometrial carcinoma. In: *Endometrial Carcinoma and its*

Precursors (eds L. Mencaglia, R.F. Valle, J. Lurain), p. 2. Isis Medical Media, Oxford. Adapted from Armstrong, B.K., Doll, R. (1975) Environmental factors and cancer incidence and mortality in different countries with special reference to dietary practices. *Int J Cancer* **15** : 617.

41 Cervical neoplasia

Figure 41.1: Coleman, D.V., Evans, D.M.D. (1998) *Biopsy Pathology and Cytology of the Cervix*. Chapman & Hall, London.

Figure 41.2: Walboomers, J.M.M., de Roda Husman, A-M, van den Brule, A.J.C., Snijders, P.J.F., Meijer, C.J.L.M. (1994) Detection of genital human papillomavirus infections: critical review of methods and prevalence studies in relation to cervical cancer. In: *Human Papillomaviruses and Cervical Cancer* (eds P.L. Stern, M.A. Stanley), p. 61. Oxford University Press, Oxford.

42 Sexually transmitted diseases

Figure 42.1: Dallabetta, G., Hook, E.W., III (1987) Gonococcal infections. *Infect Dis Clin N Amer* **1** : 1, 28.

Figure 42.2: Batteiger, B.E., Jones, R.B. (1987) Chlamydial infections. *Infect Dis Clin N Amer* **1** : 1, 58.

Table 42.1: Arrand, J.R. (1994) Molecular genetics of human papillomaviruses. In: *Human Papillomaviruses and Cervical Cancer* (eds P.L. Stern, M.A. Stanley), pp. 28–40. Oxford University Press, Oxford.

1 The pituitary gland

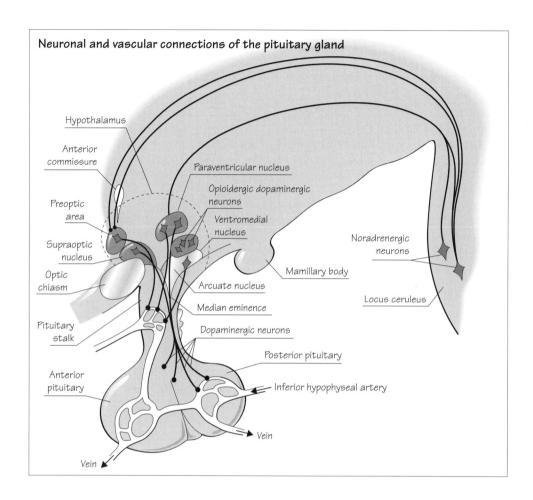

Neuronal and vascular connections of the pituitary gland

Hypothalamus

Anterior commissure

Preoptic area

Supraoptic nucleus

Optic chiasm

Pituitary stalk

Anterior pituitary

Paraventricular nucleus

Opioidergic dopaminergic neurons

Ventromedial nucleus

Arcuate nucleus

Median eminence

Dopaminergic neurons

Mamillary body

Noradrenergic neurons

Locus ceruleus

Posterior pituitary

Inferior hypophyseal artery

Vein

Vein

Structure and function

There are three lobes to the pituitary gland (hypophysis). The **anterior lobe** (adenohypophysis) is derived embryologically from endoderm lining the dorsal pharynx, which forms an outpocketing known as Rathke's pouch. The **posterior lobe** (neurohypophysis) is much smaller and derived embryologically from neuroectoderm. A small intermediate lobe (pars intermedia) which lies between the anterior and posterior lobes is actually a subdivision of the anterior lobe. Importantly, the embryologic anlage of the pituitary gland is derived from neural crest cells.

The pituitary is connected to the brain via a small stalk of tissue known as the pituitary stalk or infundibulum. The posterior pituitary serves as a storage site for two hormones made in the hypothalamus, oxytocin and arginine vasopressin (also known as antidiuretic hormone, ADH). Axons from large cell (magnocellular) neurons in the anterior hypothalamus travel into the posterior pituitary through the posterior part of the stalk. Hormones synthesized in the neuronal cell bodies of these hypothalamic cells travel down these axons where they are then stored in the posterior pituitary. The anterior pituitary produces tropic hormones under the regulatory control of the hypothalamus. Neuroendocrine signals from the hypothalamus travel through rich vascular connections surrounding the pituitary stalk. Axons from small cell (parvocellular) neurons in the hypothalamus end in the precapillary space of the primary portal system that originates at the base of the hypothalamus. Blood flowing through this highly vascular plexus delivers the trophic signals to the pituitary gland.

There are five small cell types in the anterior pituitary that are associated with trophic hormone production: gonadotropes, lactotropes, somatotropes, thyrotropes and corticotropes. These specific cell types are responsible for production and secretion of: **follicle-stimulating hormone (FSH)** and **luteinizing hormone (LH)**; **prolactin**; **growth hormone**; **thyroid-stimulating hormone (TSH)**; and **adreno-corticotropic hormone (ACTH)**, respectively. Histologically, the thyrotropes and gonadotropes resemble each other rather closely. This is because their secretory products, LH, FSH and TSH, are all glycoprotein hormones (Chapter 2) which stain with carbohydrate-sensitive chemicals. LH and FSH are produced by one cell type, consistent with their coupled secretion and regulation by a single releasing factor.

Control of the pituitary gland is largely through the hypothalamus, although pituitary cells themselves are directly sensitive to feedback mechanisms. The hypothalamic nuclei associated with reproduction include the supraoptic, paraventricular, arcuate, ventromedial and suprachiasmatic nuclei. Neurons in two less well defined areas, the medial anterior hypothalamus and the medial preoptic areas, are also involved. The magnocellular neurons, which project into the posterior pituitary and produce the hormones vasopressin and oxytocin, originate in the supraoptic and paraventricular nuclei. The parvocellular neurons are found in the paraventricular, arcuate and ventromedial nuclei and the periventricular and medial preoptic areas. The parvocellular neurons produce regulatory peptides that control gonadotrope, lactotrope, somatotrope, thyrotrope and corticotrope cell function.

Cells in the hypothalamic nuclei that regulate the pituitary have several functions. They receive signals from higher centers in the brain, they generate neural signals of their own and they have a neuroendocrine function. The areas of the brain that connect to the hypothalamic nuclei involved with reproduction are the locus ceruleus, the medulla and pons, the midbrain raphe, the olfactory bulb, the limbic system (amygdala and hippocampus), the piriform cortex and the retina. Multiple neurotransmitters are involved in the neural connections to and from the mediobasal hypothalamus. These include noradrenergic projections from the medulla, pons and locus ceruleus, serotenergic projections from the midbrain raphe and dopaminergic neurons from the limbic system. The retinal connection to the hypothalamus mediates visual influences on neuroendocrine rhythms through melatonin. Endogenous opioids also influence hypothalamic function.

The intrinsic **neural signals** relevant to reproduction that are generated within the hypothalamus itself arise from the **pulse generator** for gonadotropin-releasing hormone (GnRH) and from dopaminergic neurons that project into the median eminence of the hypothalamus. At baseline, GnRH is secreted in pulses with a frequency of one pulse per hour. Electrical recordings from the mediobasal hypothalamus reveal a synchronous increase in neuronal activity that corresponds to each LH pulse. In addition to the dopaminergic signals traveling from the hypothalamus to the pituitary stalk, there are dopaminergic neurons projecting from the hypothalamus back to the limbic system.

The **neuroendocrine signals** generated within the hypothalamus are the peptide releasing factors that travel through the hypothalamic–pituitary portal system to their site of action in the pituitary gland. **GnRH** is the key trophic hormone for regulating gonadotrope cell function and hence, reproduction (Chapter 2). **Thyrotropin-releasing hormone (TRH)** and **prolactin inhibitory factor (PIF)**, which also play roles in reproductive regulation, are described below. The remaining hypothalamic neuroendocrine peptides which control GH and ACTH secretion do not appear to be directly related to reproduction.

Prolactin is unique among the pituitary hormones in that it is under tonic inhibitory control by the hypothalamus. Prolactin inhibitory factor is none other than the neurotransmitter, dopamine, which is secreted by the hypothalamic tuberoinfundibular neurons. Prolactin is also unique among the pituitary hormones in that its secretion is not regulated by classic feedback loops involving its target organs. Instead, prolactin secretion is controlled by local autocrine and paracrine factors, neurotransmitters and peripherally produced steroid hormones. The two major positive stimuli for prolactin secretion are TRH and estradiol. TRH acts within the pituitary while estrogen is active in both the hypothalamus and pituitary. Other stimuli for prolactin secretion include serotonin, opioids, oxytocin, histamine, neurotensin and substance P at the level of the hypothalamus, and GnRH, vasoactive intestinal peptide (VIP) and angiotensin II at the level of the pituitary. The main reproductive function of prolactin is initiation and maintenance of lactation (Chapter 20). Prolactin also plays a role in immune function, much like growth hormone, with which it shares significant structural similarities.

Thyroid disorders are very common during the reproductive years, especially in women. While few of these originate within the hypothalamus or pituitary, under- and overactivity of the thyroid gland can interfere with reproductive function. The two mechanisms by which abnormal amounts of circulating thyroid hormone could affect reproductive function are either through a direct effect upon peripheral cells whose genes contain thyroid response elements or through the action of TRH on prolactin secretion. Most thyroid disease occurs because of autoimmune stimulation or destruction of the gland itself, leaving the hypothalamic pituitary axis intact. Women with underactive thyroid glands have elevated levels of TRH and TSH and women with overactive thyroid glands have virtually undetectable TRH and TSH because of the negative feedback of thyroxine on TSH secretion. TSH secretion, like that of the gonadotropins, is under hypothalamic regulation by its releasing hormone, TRH. Hypothyroid women will have elevated TRH levels because of the inadequate amount of circulating thyroxine to suppress TRH and hence TSH. As mentioned above, TRH is a very potent stimulant for prolactin release by the pituitary. Elevated levels of circulating prolactin are associated with menstrual irregularities (Chapter 28).

The posterior pituitary hormones, oxytocin and vasopressin-ADH, are cyclic nona-peptides secreted by the neurons of the supraoptic and paraventricular nuclei. Their identification and synthesis in the early 1950s represented the first concrete evidence of an endocrine function of the hypothalamus. Oxytocin has effects on uterine smooth muscle, on special myoepithelial cells in the breast and perhaps on the smooth muscle in the ejaculatory tract in men. Vasopressin-ADH has its largest effects on vascular smooth muscle and on the collecting duct of the kidney where it acts to regulate intravascular volume and osmolality. Vasopressin-ADH may also play a role in sexual arousal.

Circadian rhythms

In humans, the vital functions of the body change from day to night with a 24-h periodicity. This rhythm is known as the circadian rhythm and is entrained by environmental cues. The most important of these cues is **melatonin** secretion by the pineal gland. Melatonin is synthesized from serotonin by two enzymes known as N-acetyltransferase (NAT) and hydroxyindole-O-methyltransferase (HIOMT). Darkness activates melatonin secretion and light inhibits it. Light signals are transmitted to the pineal gland via a neural pathway that goes through a **circadian oscillator in the hypothalamus,** down the spinal cord and through the superior cervical ganglion to the pineal gland. The final neural input is a β-adrenergic sympathetic synapse. The dark-induced release of norepinephrine onto the pinealocytes activates β-adrenergic receptors that are coupled to cyclic adenosine monophosphate (cAMP) and NAT activity, thereby increasing melatonin secretion. Nocturnal melatonin secretion is associated with sleepiness, decreased core temperature and heart rate, and increased prolactin release. Melatonin has been implicated in the regulation of seasonal variations in fertility in regions with stark contrasts in day length. In the Arctic and Scandinavia, summer days are 20 h long and winter nights equally long. Melatonin concentrations are highest and conception rates are lowest during the months with the longest nights. The site of action for melatonin appears to be the hypothalamic suprachiasmatic nucleus where it inhibits metabolic activity.

2 Gonadotropins

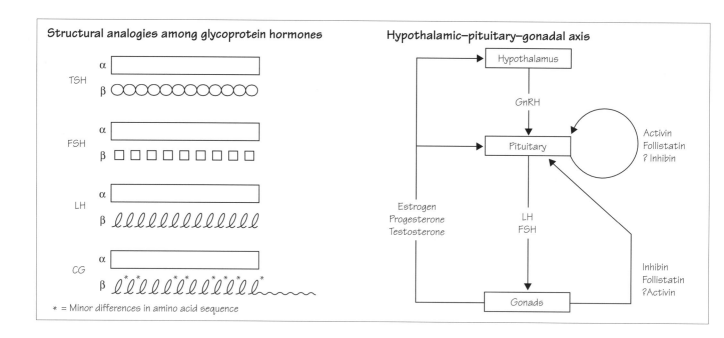

Structural analogies among glycoprotein hormones

* = Minor differences in amino acid sequence

Hypothalamic–pituitary–gonadal axis

Structure of LH and FSH

The pituitary gland produces two gonadotropins, **luteinizing hormone (LH)** and **follicle-stimulating hormone (FSH)** which are critical for gonadal function and reproduction in humans. Together with thyroid-stimulating hormone (TSH), LH and FSH form a major group of anterior pituitary hormones known as the glycoprotein hormones. Growth hormone and prolactin form a second group of structurally related hormones, and corticotropin, lipotropin, melanotropin and the endorphins, comprise the third group.

LH, FSH and TSH are structurally similar in that they are formed by two different, non-covalently bound protein subunits called α and β. The pregnancy-specific gonadotropin, human chorionic gonadotropin (hCG), is a fourth glycoprotein formed of α and β chains. The α subunit for all four hormones is identical within a group. The β subunit of each hormone is different and confers specificity on the molecule composed of the αβ units. The β chains for LH and hCG are structurally quite similar with 82% homology. Carbohydrate side chains on both the α and β chains of LH, hCG and FSH confer additional structural specificity. The carbohydrate chains also influence clearance, most notably with the hCG molecule. The β chain of hCG has a 24 amino acid extension at the C-terminus that contains four additional O-linked polysaccharides. This sugar-laden 'tail' dramatically slows the clearance of hCG; by prolonging its half-life, the effects of small amounts of the glycoprotein are dramatically enhanced. This characteristic is very important in early pregnancy recognition and maintenance (Chapters 16 and 17).

Regulation of FSH and LH

The biosynthesis and secretion of FSH and LH are tightly controlled within the reproductive cycle. Gonadotrope function is modulated by hypothalamic factors (**gonadotropin-releasing hormone, GnRH**),

pituitary factors (**activin, inhibin and follistatin**) and gonadal feedback (steroids and peptides). There are multiple ways in which FSH and LH can be regulated, including gene transcription, mRNA stabilization, rate of protein subunit synthesis, post-translational glycosylation and changes in the number of gonadotropin-secreting cells.

The hypothalamic decapeptide, **GnRH**, is synthesized within both the arcuate nucleus of the medial basal hypothalamus and the preoptic area of the anterior hypothalamus. GnRH is transported down the axons of these specialized neuroendocrine cells through the median eminence of the hypothalamus where it is released into the portal blood system that bathes the anterior pituitary (Chapter 1). GnRH is normally released in a pulsatile fashion rather than continuously. The 'pulse generator' appears to reside within the median basal hypothalamus and may be the GnRH-secreting neurons themselves. Pulsatile GnRH release stimulates gonadotropin expression whereas continuous GnRH inhibits gonadotrope function. Pulse frequency is most rapid in the early follicular phase, slightly slower in the late follicular phase and slowest in the luteal phase of the female menstrual cycle. The pulse frequency of GnRH release controls gonadotropin synthesis and secretion in an as yet unknown fashion. In general, rapid pulse frequencies favor LH secretion and slower pulse frequencies favor FSH. The relationship between pulse frequency and LH and FSH secretion appears to exist in both women and men.

Inhibin and **activin** are closely related peptides produced by the ovary, testes, pituitary gland and placenta that influence gonadotrope function. As suggested by their names, inhibin decreases gonadotrope function and activin stimulates it. Inhibin and activin are closely related peptides formed from common α and β subunits. Inhibin is formed of one α subunit linked to either of two highly homologous β subunits to form inhibin A ($\alpha\beta_A$) or inhibin B ($\alpha\beta_B$). Activin is composed of three combinations of the β subunits: activin A ($\beta_A\beta_A$), activin AB ($\beta_A\beta_B$) and activin B ($\beta_B\beta_B$). Activin is a member of the transforming growth factor β (TGF-β) superfamily of growth and differentiation factors that include TGF-β, Müllerian-inhibiting substance (MIS) and bone morphogenic proteins. It is not known if the different isoforms of inhibin and activin have divergent functions.

Follistatin is structurally unrelated to either inhibin or activin. It is a highly glycosylated peptide which also inhibits gonadotrope function but at one-third the potency of inhibin.

All three of these peptides have their major influence on the expression of the FSH-β gene. Inhibin appears to be the most biologically important of the three peptides in the regulation of the gene whose activity it suppresses directly. The other two peptides appear to act through locally released second messengers or autocrine peptides within the pituitary cells. Activin B stimulates FSH release. The activins are also active at the level of the gonad where they increase the activity of the enzyme aromatase in the ovary and stimulate proliferation of spermatogonia in the testes.

The overall effect of the **gonadal steroids** is to inhibit FSH and LH synthesis and secretion. Estrogen, androgen and progesterone receptors are present in the gonadotropin-secreting cells and in some neurons in the hypothalamus. The gonadal steroids appear to affect the transcription rate of the genes coding for FSH-β, LH-β and the common α subunit. Steroid hormone receptors do not appear to be present in the GnRH-containing cells of the arcuate nucleus; however, there is some evidence that steroids can act at the level of the hypothalamic pulse generator.

There is one important exception to the generally inhibitory effect of gonadal steroids on gonadotrope function. Estrogen exerts a positive feedback on gonadotropin secretion that is critical to produce the mid-cycle LH surge in women (Chapter 13). This effect requires a sustained elevation in circulating estradiol that lasts for about 48 h. Estrogen appears to stimulate both gonadotropin gene expression in the pituitary and GnRH pulse frequency in the hypothalamus.

Mechanism of action of gonadotropins

The **receptors** for the glycoprotein hormones are located in the plasma membrane of their target cells in the gonads. There is an FSH receptor and an LH receptor that also bind the closely related hCG molecule. Both these receptors are normally present in very low concentrations on the cell surface but have high specificity and affinity for their ligands. The interactions between the glycoprotein dimer and the receptor lead to a conformational change in the receptor. This then leads to the activation of a membrane-associated **G protein-coupled signaling system**. Other important members of the G protein receptor family include receptors for GnRH and for α-adrenergic, β-adrenergic and dopaminergic compounds. Receptor binding and receptor activation with intracellular signal activation are distinct events in this receptor superfamily and may be differentially affected by different disease processes.

G proteins are a subset of regulatory guanosine triphosphate (GTP)-binding proteins that activate adenylate cyclase and increase intracellular cAMP production. The conformational change induced by binding of the gonadotropin on the surface results in the replacement of an intracellular subunit of the G-protein with GTP. The dissociated G protein subunit ($G_{s\alpha}$) then activates adenylate cyclase to produce cAMP. Increased cAMP activates the intracellular protein kinase A pathway

which in turn modulates the function of a number of cell processes by protein phosphorylation. In the ovary and testes, it is the increase in cAMP that is responsible for gonadal steroidogenesis and gametogenesis (Chapter 3).

Although the cAMP pathway is the principal mediator of both FSH and LH receptor activity, it would appear that activation of the protein kinase C system can also occur. This involves activation of a different G protein subunit, G_q, by LH/hCG binding to the LH receptor. G_q then activates phospholipase C which produces two intracellular messengers, 1,2-diacylglycerol (DAG) and inositol triphosphate ($InsP_3$) from membrane lipids. DAG activates protein kinase C and $InsP_3$ releases calcium sequestered in the endoplasmic reticulum into the intracellular space.

In addition to activating specific intracellular processes, binding of the gonadotropin to its receptor also initiates another regulatory function called **desensitization**. In the first phase of desensitization, the receptor becomes 'uncoupled' from its receptor activity so that it no longer activates adenylate cyclase. In the second phase of desensitization, the degradation rate for the receptors is increased. This slower process is called 'down-regulation'. Desensitization reduces the cell's responsiveness to ongoing stimulation.

Both LH and FSH receptors are present on the plasma membranes of granulosa cells in the ovary and Sertoli cells in the testes. Ovarian thecal cells and testicular Leydig cells only have LH receptors. In addition to regulating steroidogenesis and gametogenesis, both of the gonadotropins regulate expression of their own receptors in a dose-dependent fashion. FSH also induces LH/hCG receptor formation in granulosa and Sertoli cells.

A carefully defined sequence of hormonal changes is necessary for normal follicular development and ovulation in the ovary (Chapter 13). Initiation of follicular growth occurs independently from gonadotropin stimulation; however, unless gonadotropins are present, these follicles will rapidly undergo atresia. FSH causes granulosa cell proliferation and estrogen biosynthesis around the developing follicles. Theca cells lack FSH receptors and only respond to LH; LH increases the production of androgen precursors in the thecal cells (Chapter 3). FSH induces the enzyme, aromatase, within the granulosa cells. Aromatase converts the androgens produced in the theca cells to estrogens in the granulosa cells. FSH also increases inhibin production by the granulosa cells prior to ovulation.

Once ovulation has occured, the theca cells from the follicle are converted to a corpus luteum. Progesterone production by the corpus luteum is stimulated by LH. LH increases the cellular uptake of both low-density lipoprotein (LDL) cholesterol by induction of LDL receptors and the two rate-limiting enzyme complexes, P450cc and 3β-hydroxysteroid dehydrogenase, necessary for progesterone synthesis. Maintenance of steroid production by the corpus luteum is LH dependent; however, the finite 14-day life span of the corpus luteum does not appear to be related to a decrease in LH stimulation. The factor(s) responsible for the demise of the corpus luteum are unknown. As the function of the corpus luteum wanes near the end of the cycle, synthesis of inhibin, estrogen and progesterone decreases and production of FSH by the pituitary increases. This next wave of FSH production 'rescues' developing follicles from atresia.

In the male, FSH stimulates spermatogenesis within the seminiferous epithelium and production of testosterone and inhibin by the Sertoli cells. LH stimulates testosterone production by the Leydig cells.

3 Steroid hormone biosynthesis

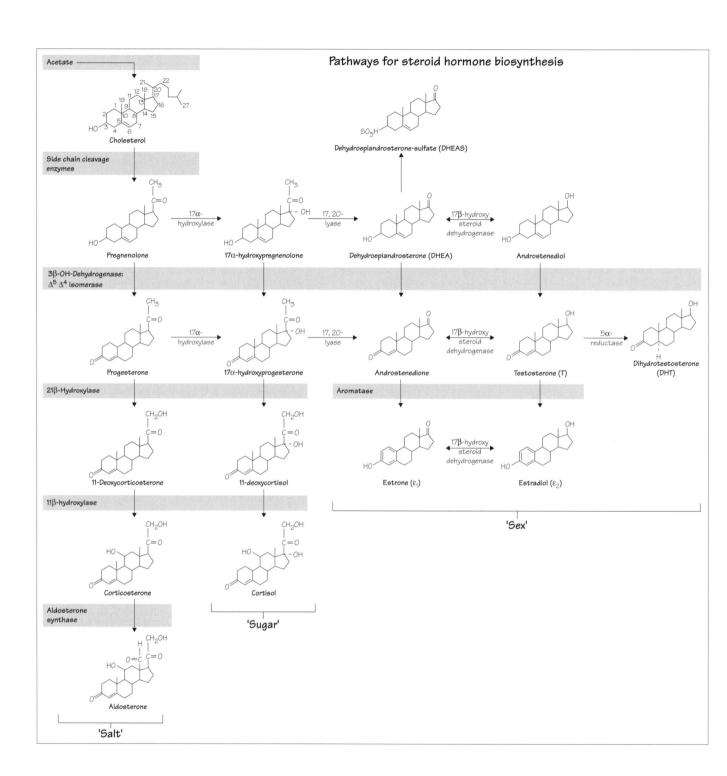

Pathways for steroid hormone biosynthesis

Cholesterol and the steroid production pathway

Cholesterol is the building block of steroid hormones. All steroid-producing organs with the exception of the placenta can synthesize cholesterol from acetate; however, under most circumstances, local synthesis cannot meet demand and circulating cholesterol must be used. The major carriers of cholesterol in the bloodstream are the **low-density lipoproteins (LDLs)**. LDL is removed from the blood by surface receptors on steroidogenic cells that recognize specific surface proteins on LDL called apoproteins. Once in the cell, cholesterol is carried through a sequence of enzymatic changes to produce a final product that belongs to one of the major classes of steroid hormones: progestins, androgens, estrogens (sex), glucocorticoids (sugar) and mineralocorticoids (salt). All steroid-producing tissues use a common sequence of precursor molecules and enzymes. Tissue specificity is conferred by the presence or absence of specific enzymes in the sequence. The gonads differ from the adrenal glands in that ovaries and testes do not express the 21-hydroxylase or 11β-hydroxylase enzymes that are necessary to produce corticosteroids. Therefore, the gonads only produce three classes of steroids: progestins, androgens and estrogens.

Most of the steroidogenic enzymes are members of the **cytochrome P450 class of oxidases**. A single mitochondrial protein P450scc, the cholesterol side chain cleavage enzyme, mediates all steps between cholesterol and pregnenolone. This step is rate limiting for the entire steroid pathway. It is the major site of trophic hormone stimulation. Genetic mutations of P450scc are very rare and usually lethal because no steroid hormones can form.

During steroidogenesis from cholesterol, the number of total carbon atoms can only decrease. Progestins have 21 carbons (C-21); androgens, 19 carbons (C-19); and estrogens, 18 carbons (C-18). Thus progestins are obligatory precursors of both androgens and estrogens. Likewise, androgens are obligatory precursors of estrogens.

Once pregnenolone is formed, steroid production can proceed down one of two paths through either progesterone or 17α-hydroxypregnenolone. All but two of the enzymes responsible for producing the steroid hormones are packaged together with other members of the P450 system within the endoplasmic reticulum. The biosynthetic units are very tightly linked together, thereby ensuring that very few of the steroid intermediates leave the cell. This packaging is also highly efficient in that it can convert an entire class of steroids to another. Thus, 17,20-desmolase will convert all progestins to androgens and aromatase will convert all androgens but dihydrotestosterone (DHT) to estrogens.

Sites of production
Ovary
In the ovary, steroid production occurs in a **two-cell system**. Theca cells produce androgens that then diffuse into the granulosa cells where they are converted to estrogens. Trophic hormones regulate specific steps in the sex steroid cascade. Theca cells respond to **luteinizing hormone (LH)** by increasing the number of LDL receptors and hence cholesterol entry into the cells. LH also stimulates P450scc activity and androgens are produced in increased quantities. Androgens then diffuse into the granulosa cells where **follicle-stimulating hormone (FSH)** induces aromatase activity, thereby increasing the conversion of androgens to estrogens. The single aromatase gene has many promoter sites responsive to cytokines, cyclic nucleotides, gonadotropins, glucocorticoids and growth factors.

Testes
In the testes, androgen production occurs largely in the Leydig cells under the influence of LH. Androgens produced in the Leydig cells either enter the blood stream directly or diffuse into nearby Sertoli cells. Sertoli cells can convert androgens to estrogens or reduce them to dihydrotestosterone via 5α-reductase. Steroid production in the testes very much parallels that in the ovary because of the common embryonic origins of specific cell types within the differentiated gonads (Chapter 5.2).

Adrenals
Sex hormone production by the adrenals occurs largely as a by-product of corticosteroid biosynthesis. The contribution of adrenal sex steroids to the total pool of circulating sex steroids is usually small with several important exceptions. The ovaries of postmenopausal women no longer produce steroid hormones; thus adrenal androgen production can be clinically significant in some women. In pregnancy, the placenta cannot synthesize cholesterol from acetate and relies on adrenal androgens of both maternal and fetal origin to make estrogen.

Inherited defects in any of the enzymes involved in steroidogenesis except for P450scc are associated with clinical syndromes that result either from the build-up of a precursor or from the absence of a key steroid hormone end product. For example, an inherited deficiency of the enzyme 21-hydroxylase in the adrenal will lead to a deficiency in cortisol production. This deficiency feeds back to stimulate enhanced production of precursor progestins, some of which will flow down the androgen biosynthetic pathways. In a female fetus, the increase in androgen will lead to masculinization of the external genitalia, a condition known as congenital adrenal hyperplasia syndrome (Chapter 25). Similarly, disorders of male sexual differentiation and development can occur with genetic defects in androgen production (Chapter 24).

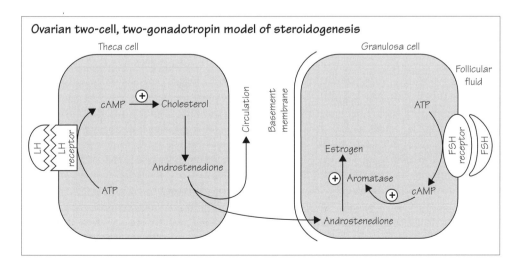

Ovarian two-cell, two-gonadotropin model of steroidogenesis

4 Steroid hormone mechanism of action and metabolism

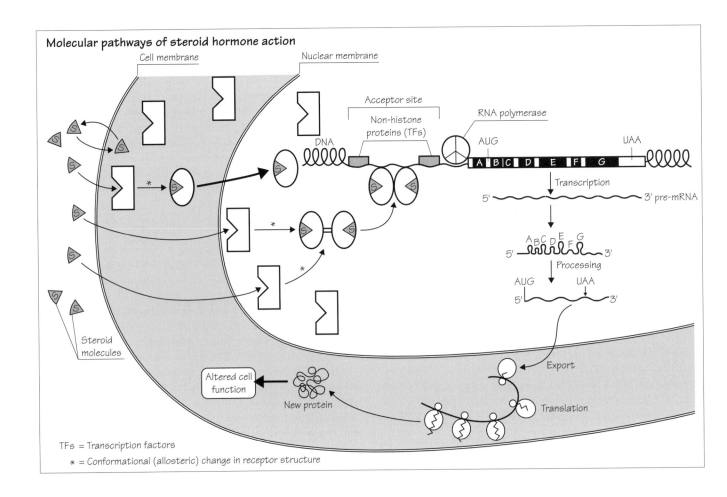

Molecular pathways of steroid hormone action

Cell membrane

Nuclear membrane

Acceptor site

Non-histone proteins (TFs)

RNA polymerase

DNA

AUG

UAA

A B C D E F G

Transcription

5' — 3' pre-mRNA

A B C D E F G

5' — 3'

Processing

AUG UAA

5' — 3'

Export

Translation

Steroid molecules

Altered cell function

New protein

TFs = Transcription factors

* = Conformational (allosteric) change in receptor structure

Mechanisms of steroid action

The basic mechanism of action of steroid hormones is induction of new protein synthesis in their target cells. These proteins may be hormones themselves or other molecules important to cell function such as enzymes. It is the new proteins synthesized that are ultimately responsible for steroid hormone activity.

Once a steroid hormone is secreted by its endocrine gland of origin, 95–98% of it circulates in the bloodstream bound to a specific transport protein. The remaining 2–5% is free to diffuse into all cells. Once in the cell, the steroid can only produce responses in cells that have **specific intracellular receptors** for that hormone. Specific receptor binding is key to the action of steroids in their target tissues. Thus, estrogen receptors are found in target cells specific to females such as the uterus, breast and brain. Facial hair follicles and penile erectile tissue contain androgen receptors. Glucocorticoid receptors are found in all cells because they are necessary to regulate metabolism and stress.

In the cell, each of the major classes of sex steroids, androgens, estrogens and progestins acts through a common sequence of events which includes: (i) transfer of the steroid into the nucleus followed by receptor binding; (ii) allosteric conformational changes in receptor structure which convert the receptor from an inactive to an active form;

(iii) binding of the steroid–receptor complex to regulatory elements on DNA; (iv) transcription and synthesis of new mRNA; and (v) translation of mRNA with new protein synthesis in the cell. Glucocorticoids and mineralocorticoids differ in that they first bind to their receptors in the cytoplasm and are then transported to the nucleus where they bind to the DNA.

There are three important structural domains in each steroid hormone receptor that correspond to the molecule's three functions: (i) steroid hormone binding; (ii) DNA binding; and (iii) gene transcription. Molecular cloning of the copy DNA for all steroid hormone receptors has demonstrated remarkable structural similarities among them. In addition, the receptors for thyroid hormone, vitamin D and vitamin A also have similar DNA binding domains. Together with the sex hormone receptors, these receptors form a 'superfamily' of nuclear receptors of which the thyroid hormone and vitamin A and D receptors are thought to be the most evolutionarily primitive. These three receptors are highly conserved because of their importance in early embryonic development. The more evolutionarily recent glucocorticoid and progesterone receptors regulate acute metabolic changes in highly differentiated cells.

Expression of genes regulated by steroid hormones is controlled by four specific elements called (i) promoters, (ii) steroid-responsive enhancers, (iii) silencers and (iv) hormone-independent enhancers. The steroid-responsive enhancers are the DNA binding sites for the activated steroid–receptor complexes and are known as steroid response elements (SREs). SREs are a very important component of these genes as they confer the steroid specificity on the gene.

Agonists and antagonists

Much of the pharmacology and physiology of steroid hormone action has been learned from biochemical studies of steroid receptors. Steroid hormone potency depends on a combination of the affinity of the receptor for the hormone or drug and the efficiency of the allosterically activated hormone–receptor complex in regulating gene transcription. Molecules with high affinities lead to prolonged occupancy of the SRE and sustained gene transcription. Such molecules act as agonists for the parent compound. Conversely, molecules that occupy the steroid receptor in a way that allows them to bind to the SRE but prevents RNA polymerase from coupling with factors necessary for gene transcription will act as antagonists to the parent compound. An example of a compound with mixed agonist/antagonist properties is the drug tamoxifen. **Tamoxifen** is an antiestrogen that acts as a potent antagonist to the estrogen receptor in breast tissue and as an agonist in uterus and bone. Such tissue-specific effects are dependent upon the specific silencers and hormone-independent enhancers present in each tissue. Another widely used agonist/antagonist is the non-steroidal drug clomiphene that can be used to induce ovulation. **Clomiphene** unproductively occupies estrogen receptors in the hypothalamus thereby creating a local hypo-estrogenic state. GnRH pulse frequency increases and follicle-stimulating hormone (FSH) production is stimulated. FSH increases ovarian production of estrogen that acts locally to recruit follicles for ovulation. When the clomiphene is stopped, the hypothalamus again senses the high concentrations of circulating estrogen from the ovaries and an ovulatory luteinizing hormone (LH) surge occurs (Chapter 13).

Steroids in the circulation

Steroid hormones are transported in the bloodstream bound to specific proteins. Most of the testosterone and estradiol is bound to a β globulin known as **sex hormone-binding globulin (SHBG)**. Another 30% is loosely bound to albumin, leaving only 1–2% unbound and capable of entering cells. SHBG binds all estrogens and androgens to varying degrees; less than 10% of any steroid is free in the bloodstream. Pregnancy, estrogen and hyperthyroidism all increase SHBG synthesis. Androgens, progestins, corticoids and growth hormone all decrease SHBG. Weight gain can also decrease SHBG through an insulin-mediated effect on its synthesis. Changes in the concentration of SHBG will affect the amount of free, unbound steroid by the law of mass action. Thus, these changes in SHBG will affect the biologic action of the steroids by altering the amount available to cells.

Progesterone is carried in the blood by a glycoprotein, cortico-steroid-binding globulin (CBG), which also carries glucocorticoids. CBG is also known as transcortin.

Steroid metabolism

Androgens are obligatory precursors of all steroid hormones except for progestins. Therefore they are made by each of the steroid-producing tissues including the testes, ovary and adrenal gland. The major circulating androgen in men is testosterone that is produced by the testes. **Testosterone is the most potent androgen**. Its hormonal action is produced either directly through binding to the androgen receptor or indirectly by **conversion to dihydrotestosterone (DHT)** within the target tissue. Testosterone acts directly during sexual differentiation of the internal genital tract in male fetuses (Chapter 5.3) and on skeletal muscle to promote growth. DHT is active in differentiating and maintaining the external genitalia and secondary sexual characteristics such as facial and pubic hair. Other major circulating androgens in men include androstenedione, androstenediol, dehydroepiandrosterone (DHEA) and dehydroepiandrosterone sulfate (DHEA-S).

All of the above androgens, including testosterone and DHT, can be found in the circulation of women. With the exception of androstenedione, the concentrations of the androgens are considerably less in women than in men. Androstenedione is unique in that only about 4% of it is bound to SHBG in the circulation in women. The remainder is bound more loosely to albumin. Circulating androstenedione functions largely as a prohormone and is converted within target tissues to testosterone, estrone and estradiol.

Estradiol (E_2) is the major estrogen secreted by the ovary. Estrone (E_1) is also secreted by the ovary in significant amounts. Estriol (E_3), by contrast, is not produced in the ovary at all. Estriol is produced from estradiol and estrone in peripheral tissues and from androgen in the placenta and is considered a less active 'metabolite' of the more potent estrogens. Direct conversion of androgens into estrone can occur in skin and adipose tissue. Conversion of androgens to estrone in obese women can be the source of large amounts of estrogen, given that the daily production of androstenedione is 10 times higher than estradiol.

The adrenal gland is the source of significant amounts of sex steroids in both men and women. Adrenal production of androgens follows a circadian rhythm that parallels cortisol secretion. Androstenedione, DHEA and DHEA-S are the major circulating androgens of adrenal origin. Adrenal androgens assume an important role in the postmenopausal woman where they can serve as important precursors to estrogens.

The major progestin in the circulation is **progesterone**. The ovary, testes, placenta and adrenal gland produce progesterone. 17-Hydroxyprogesterone of adrenal and ovarian origin also circulates. Both progestins are largely bound by transcortin.

Steroid excretion

Steroids are excreted in urine and bile. Prior to elimination, most active steroids are conjugated as either sulfates or glucuronides. Some sulfated conjugates such as DHEA-S are actively secreted and can serve as precursors in target tissues that have the enzymes to hydrolyze the ester bonds.

5 Embryology of the reproductive tract

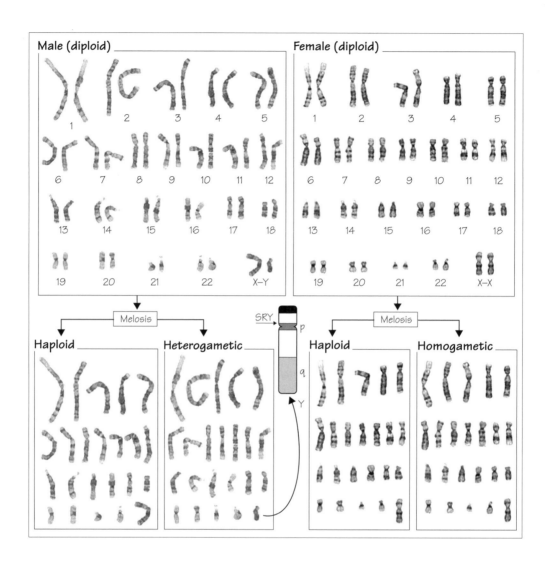

1 ROLE OF SEX CHROMATIN IN REPRODUCTIVE DEVELOPMENT

In humans, like all other mammalian species, the female is the homogametic sex, meaning that all gametes produced by a genetic female have the same 22X chromosomal constitution. The human female is also the 'fundamental' or undifferentiated phenotypic sex. In the absence of specific factors regulated by a single gene on the Y chromosome, embryos will develop a female phenotype. This is true of all mammals and occurs because of the large amount of placental estrogen bathing embryos of both genetic sexes.

The male is the heterogametic sex that produces gametes with both 22X and 22Y chromosome complements. The male is also the 'differentiated' phenotypic sex. Individuals carrying a Y chromosome or a specific piece of it will develop a testis and a male phenotype with few exceptions. **The important step in differentiation is a specific instruction from the Y chromosome telling the undifferentiated gonad to become a testis.**

The Y chromosome is much smaller than the X and very little of the DNA is available for RNA synthesis. Therefore many of the genes that control testicular development from the undifferentiated gonad are, by necessity, located on other chromosomes including autosomes and the X chromosome. The Y chromosome contains a specific, single-copy gene located in the **sex-determining region of the Y chromosome (SRY)**, which is located on the short arm of the chromosome. The sex-determining gene within SRY appears to activate genes on several other chromosomes, including autosomes and the X chromosome.

Evidence for the importance of SRY comes from both clinical and experimental research results. Examination of the DNA sequences of men with XX karyotypes and women with XY karyotypes has revealed that a single locus must be present and intact for an individual to have a testis. Absence of or damage to this DNA sequence results in ovarian development and a phenotypic female.

2 GONADAL DIFFERENTIATION

Gonadal development begins in the human at the 4th embryonic (6th menstrual) week in parallel with the formation of the ventral body wall. The first step is the migration of undifferentiated primordial germ cells from their site of formation in the yolk sac. These germ cells arise from the endoderm lining the yolk sac, detach themselves and migrate dorsally along the yolk stalk, midgut and dorsal mesentery to reach the genital ridges. The genital ridges lie on the medial aspect of the mesonephric ridge that will contribute to the developing kidney. Over the next 2 weeks the primordial germ cells mitose repeatedly, forming a vast population of precursor gametes. Failure of these germ cells to develop and populate the genital ridges will result in total failure of the gonads to develop.

Upon touching the coelomic epithelium lining the genital ridge, the germ cells cause it to differentiate into a primitive germinal epithelium. The germ cells become embedded in the primitive germinal epithelium during the process of differentiation, forming sex cords. The connection of the sex cords to the coelomic wall (gonadal surface) is maintained. The gonads at this point are histologically distinct, bipotent organs that may become testes or ovaries. Inappropriate or incomplete developmental signals at this point can result in the rare condition of true hermaphroditism.

In a genetic male, gene products directed by activation of the SRY locus on the Y chromosome now cause the undifferentiated sex cords to enlarge, split and begin to form **primitive testes**. Subepithelial mesenchyme arising between the germinal epithelium and the sex cords cuts the cords off from the gonadal surface. The **medulla**, which is the inner portion of the gonad, now houses the sex cords. The primordial germ cells within the sex cords begin to differentiate into immature sperm cells called **spermatogonia**. The supporting cord cells form precursor **Sertoli cells**.

Ovarian differentiation occurs about 2 weeks later than testicular development. Initially, the sex cords continue to proliferate while maintaining their connection with the gonadal surface. The germ cells begin to differentiate into primordial **oocytes** called oogonia within follicles. The epithelium surrounding the oogonia differentiates into **granulosa cells**. Subepithelial mesenchyme then invades the gonad and breaks up the sex cords, isolating the follicles. This mesenchyme will become the ovarian stroma. The **cortex**, or outer portion, of the gonad now houses the developing follicles.

The ovary and testes are histologically distinct by the 8th embryonic (10th menstrual) week of pregnancy. The progeny of the germinal epithelium are now apparent as Sertoli cells in the male and granulosa cells in the female. Similarities in their endocrine function in males and females stem from their common ancestry. The mesenchyme arising beneath the germinal epithelium is the anlagen of testicular interstitial cells, also known as **Leydig cells**, and ovarian stroma or **thecal cells**. Functional similarities in these two cell types also will be seen in the mature glands.

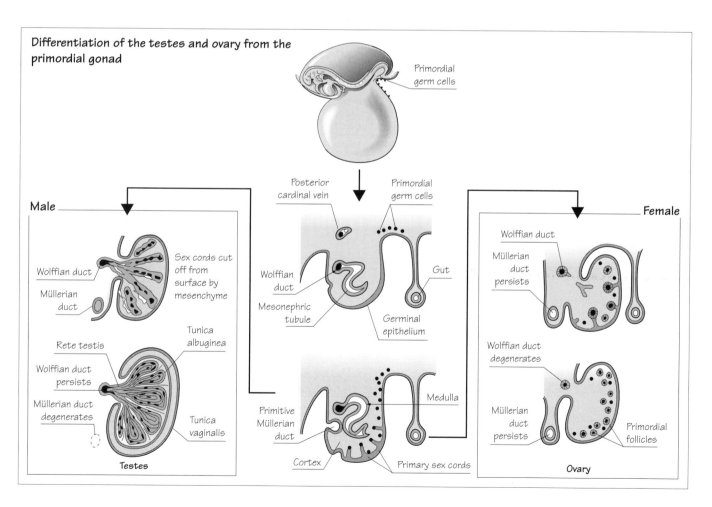

Differentiation of the testes and ovary from the primordial gonad

Primordial germ cells

Posterior cardinal vein

Primordial germ cells

Male

Female

Wolffian duct

Müllerian duct

Sex cords cut off from surface by mesenchyme

Wolffian duct

Mesonephric tubule

Gut

Germinal epithelium

Wolffian duct

Müllerian duct persists

Rete testis

Tunica albuginea

Wolffian duct persists

Müllerian duct degenerates

Tunica vaginalis

Primitive Müllerian duct

Medulla

Wolffian duct degenerates

Müllerian duct persists

Primordial follicles

Testes

Cortex

Primary sex cords

Ovary

3 PHENOTYPIC SEX DIFFERENTIATION— INTERNAL GENITALIA

Once the gonads begin to develop into either ovaries or testes, the remainder of sexual differentiation is dependent on secretory products of the testes only. In the absence of these specific testicular secretions, the phenotype that develops is totally female. Experimental data from animals and naturally occuring developmental abnormalities in humans have shown that the ovary does not contribute to the development of the uterus, Fallopian tubes or vulva.

The internal genitalia are unique in sexual development in that, unlike the gonads and external genitalia which are bipotential, separate duct systems develop into male and female structures. These internal organs of reproduction begin to develop in parallel with the urinary system and the gonad at about 4 embryonic (6 menstrual) weeks. The primordial kidney (mesonephros) is composed of tubules and a duct known as the **mesonephric or Wolffian duct**. The Wolffian duct grows out from the tubules toward the urogenital sinus. The mesonephric tubules make contact with the primitive sex cords just as the gonad begins to differentiate. Simultaneously, an inpocketing of the coelomic epithelium near the lateral edge of the mesonephric ridge forms the paramesonephric or **Müllerian duct**. Upon reaching the uro-

genital sinus, the Müllerian ducts induce the formation of a tubercle. As kidney development proceeds (metanephric stage), the mesonephric structures will become totally incorporated into the reproductive tract and lose their urinary function. The Wolffian and Müllerian ducts are the primordia from which the internal organs of reproduction will develop in the male and female, respectively. In each sex, the other duct system typically disappears by the 3rd fetal month, leaving behind only unimportant vestiges.

In the normal male embryo, the secretion of a peptide called Müllerian-inhibiting substance (MIS) occurs under the direction of SRY. MIS is a member of the transforming growth factor beta (TGF-β) superfamily of peptide hormones and is secreted by the cells destined to become Sertoli cells in the testes. MIS causes the Müllerian duct to degenerate. Testosterone formed by the testicular cells destined to become Leydig cells then directs development of the **Wolffian duct system** to form the **epididymis**, **vas deferens** and **seminal vesicles**. Testosterone production by the embryonic testes is under the control of a placental hormone called human chorionic gonadotropin (hCG) and not the hypothalamic–pituitary system.

The prostate gland forms from tissue at the base of the disappearing Müllerian tubercle (colliculus seminalis). Most of the **prostate gland** develops from the same primordial area of the urogenital sinus that

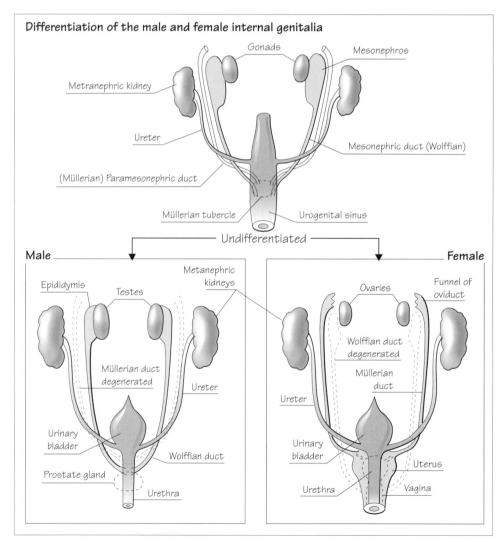

Differentiation of the male and female internal genitalia

forms the vaginal plate in the female and thus is a homolog of the upper vagina. The mesenchyme in this tissue differentiates into the peripheral zone of the prostate, under the influence of **dihydrotestosterone (DHT)** produced locally from testosterone by the enzyme 5α-reductase. The more central tissue, which may be of Wolffian derivation, forms the central and transition zones of the prostate.

In the female embryo, the absence of MIS permits the Müllerian system to persist. Upon reaching the urogenital sinus, the Müllerian ducts induce the formation of a vaginal plate which initiates the fusion of the ducts to form the body of the uterus. The Müllerian ducts will form the **Fallopian tubes**, **uterus** and **upper one-third of the vagina**. Failure of the Müllerian ducts to develop or fuse completely can cause uterine and cervical anomalies. In the absence of testosterone, the Wolffian system then regresses. A vestige of the Wolffian duct, known as Gartner's duct, persists in its length from the ovary to the hymen. Clinically apparent cysts may form anywhere along Gartner's duct.

4 PHENOTYPIC SEX DIFFERENTIATION— EXTERNAL GENITALIA

Like the primordial gonads, the anlagen of the external genitalia are bipotential. In the 8th embryonic (10th menstrual) week, a urogenital slit, a genital tubercle, two lateral genital folds and two labioscrotal swellings become apparent.

In contrast to differentiation of the internal Wolffian duct system that is testosterone dependent, the primordial external genital structures require the presence of **dihydrotestosterone** (**DHT**) to differentiate into recognizably male structures. The source of the DHT is testicular testosterone that is converted to DHT in the primordial external genitalia. In the presence of DHT, the lobes of the **prostate gland** grow out from the seminal colliculus where the urethra is developing from the bladder. The genital folds fuse to form the **penis** around the elongating urethra. The labioscrotal swellings enlarge and fuse to form the **scrotum**.

The descent of the testes from the abdomen into the scrotum is an androgen-dependent event during which the testes are pulled downward by the **gubernaculum**, a fibrous cord anchored to the developing scrotum. During development, a peritoneal fold around the Wolffian and Müllerian ducts (destined to eventually become the tunica vaginalis) connects to the genital swelling, and the gubernaculum begins to develop as a ridge under the peritoneum. The gubernaculum connecting the testis to the genital swelling does not grow as rapidly as the remainder of the embryo and hence each testis is progressively pulled down toward the developing scrotum. The testes sit just above the inguinal ring until the last three months of pregnancy at which time they complete their descent through the inguinal canal into the scrotum. After full descent of the testis, the inguinal canal narrows, thereby preventing abdominal contents from dropping into the scrotum.

Unlike differentiation of the external and internal genitalia that relies on hCG stimulation of testicular androgen production, testicular descent requires fetal gonadotropins. Disruptions in the fetal hypothalamic-pituitary-testicular axis result in failure of the testes to descend properly (cryptorchidism). Recent evidence indicates that expression of calcitonin gene-related peptide (CGRP), located within the genitofemoral nerve, might be the final common pathway by which androgens control testicular descent. MIS produced in the Sertoli cells may be involved in male gubernacular function as well.

In the female, the folds of the urogenital slit remain open. The posterior aspect of the urogenital sinus forms the **lower two-thirds of the vagina** and the anterior aspect forms the urethra. The lateral genital folds form the **labia minora** and the labioscrotal swellings form the **labia majora**. The **clitoris** forms above the urethra. The gubernaculum that forms between the edge of the Müllerian duct and the ovary becomes secondarily attached to the cornua of the uterus as it differentiates. The gubernaculum in the female becomes the ovarian and round ligaments. The tract through which the gubernaculum attaches to the labioscrotal swelling is obliterated by connective tissue shortly before birth in girls. Female phenotypic differentiation occurs in the absence of androgen and is not dependent on an ovary to proceed.

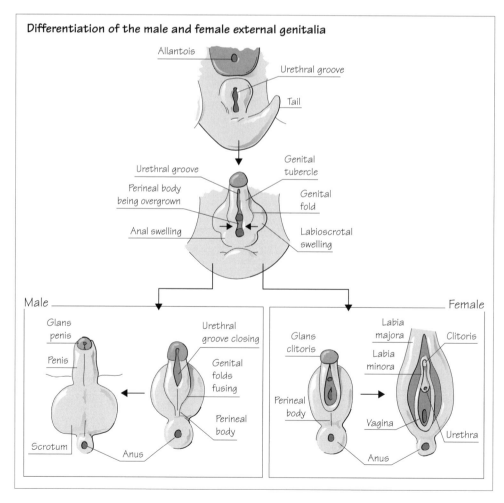

Differentiation of the male and female external genitalia

Thus, exposure to specific androgens beginning in the 5th embryonic (7th menstrual) week of pregnancy is critical to the development of a recognizable newborn male phenotype. Fetuses exposed to DHT at this time will be masculinized regardless of the genetic or gonadal sex. Conversely, a lack of androgen activity will result in a female phenotype.

Fetal sex based on the external genitalia is apparent to the experienced examiner at the end of the 12th embryonic (14th menstrual) week. Fetal sex can usually be identified on prenatal ultrasound by 16–18 menstrual weeks.

6 Gross anatomy of the male reproductive tract

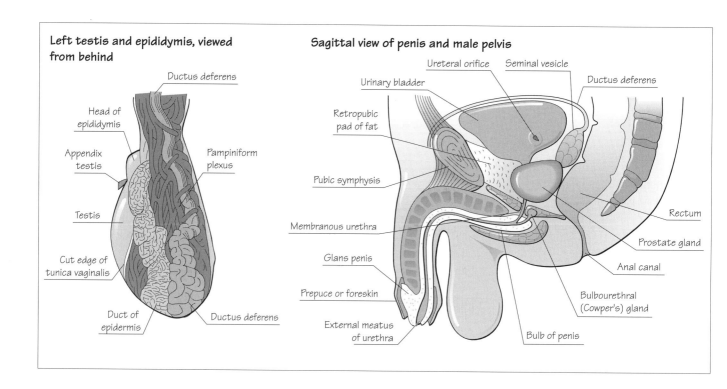

Left testis and epididymis, viewed from behind

- Ductus deferens
- Head of epididymis
- Appendix testis
- Pampiniform plexus
- Testis
- Cut edge of tunica vaginalis
- Duct of epidermis
- Ductus deferens

Sagittal view of penis and male pelvis

- Ureteral orifice
- Seminal vesicle
- Urinary bladder
- Ductus deferens
- Retropubic pad of fat
- Pubic symphysis
- Membranous urethra
- Glans penis
- Prepuce or foreskin
- External meatus of urethra
- Rectum
- Prostate gland
- Anal canal
- Bulbourethral (Cowper's) gland
- Bulb of penis

Testes and epididymis

The testes are a pair of oval, slightly flattened bodies measuring about 4 cm in length and 2.5 cm in diameter. Together with the epididymis, they lie in the scrotum, an extra-abdominal sac that lies just below the penis. The walls of the cavity in which the testes and epididymis reside are known as the **tunica vaginalis**. The tunica vaginalis forms from intra-abdominal peritoneum that migrates into the primitive scrotum during development of the male internal genitalia. After migration of the testis into the scrotum, the channel down which the testis has moved (processus vaginalis) is obliterated.

The epididymis is a comma-shaped structure that clasps the postero-lateral margin of the testes. It is formed from an irregularly twisted tube called the duct of the epididymis. The epididymal duct is about 600 cm in length. It begins at the top of the testes as the head of the epididymis and ends, after an extraordinarily tortuous course, at the tail where it becomes the vas deferens.

The arterial blood supply of the testes and epididymis is the testicular arteries that arise from the aorta just below the renal arteries. The arteries end in a dense vascular plexus called the **pampiniform plexus** which courses just under the tunica vaginalis surrounding the testes. The plexus then drains into the testicular veins. The pampiniform plexus is an important structure in temperature regulation of the testes because it can dissipate heat out of the scrotum by vasodilatation. **Like the ovarian veins, the right testicular vein empties into the inferior vena cava, and the left testicular vein into the left renal vein.** Lymphatic drainage of the testes is to the para-aortic nodes.

All the blood and lymph vessels to the testis and epididymis enter the scrotum from the abdomen through the inguinal canal bundled in a structure known as the **spermatic cord**. In addition to the blood and lymph vessels, the spermatic cord contains the **vas deferens** and any remnants of the processus vaginalis.

The testis is the site of spermatogenesis and sex steroid production in the male. The epididymis is the site of final sperm maturation. The scrotum is basically a specialized dermal pouch that protects the testis and epididymis from physical injury and aids in heat regulation of the testes. Spermatozoa are very heat sensitive; the testes and epididymis are outside the body cavity to ensure an intratesticular temperature that is lower than in the abdomen.

Vas (ductus) deferens and seminal vesicles

The vas deferens is the direct continuation of the epididymis. It is a 45-cm-long structure that begins at the lower end of the epididymis and ascends along the posterior aspect of the testis in loose coils. After leaving the back of the testis, the vas deferens traverses the spermatic cord into the abdomen. The vas deferens may be felt as a firm hard cord on the posterior aspect of the spermatic cord as it traverses the scrotum to the superficial inguinal ring. After crossing into the abdomen, the vas deferens curves medially across the external iliac artery toward the pelvis. From there, it crosses the obturator nerve and vessels and the vesicular vessels. The vas then crosses over the ureter to meet the duct of the seminal vesicle. Together they form the **ejaculatory duct** that opens into the prostatic portion of the urethra. The vas deferens dilates as it approaches the seminal vesicle; this dilated ampulla looks very much like the seminal vesicle it is about to join. The ejaculatory duct is short (2.5 cm) and lies very close to its fellow duct from the opposite side as they pass forward through the prostate.

The seminal vesicles are a pair of hollow, sacculated structures located at the base of the bladder in front of the rectum. Each vesicle is about 5 cm in length and is more intimately connected to the bladder than to the rectum. The seminal vesicles are embryological diverticula of the vas deferens and share a common blood and lymphatic supply with it.

The blood supply to the vas deferens and seminal vesicles is mainly from the inferior vesicular artery that also supplies the bladder. The artery accompanies the vas into the scrotum where it anastomoses with the testicular artery. Lymphatic drainage is to the internal and external iliac nodes.

The functions of the vas deferens and seminal vesicles are sperm transport and production of seminal fluid, respectively.

Prostate gland

The prostate is a partly glandular, partly muscular organ that surrounds the beginning of the male urethra. It is a $2 \times 3 \times 4$ cm organ that is firmly affixed by a connective tissue sheath just behind the symphysis pubis. The median lobe of the prostate, which is also known histologically as the transition zone, is the wedge-shaped portion of the gland that surrounds the urethra and separates it from the ejaculatory ducts. When hypertrophied, as it often is in elderly men, the median lobe of the prostate may cause a pressure elevation in the bladder and obstruct the flow of urine.

The anterior prostate is composed mostly of fibromuscular tissue. The glandular tissue of the prostate is situated at the sides of the urethra and immediately posterior to it. The glandular tissue is subdivided into a central and peripheral zone based on the embryology (Chapter 5.3) and histology (Chapter 7). The peripheral zone is much larger than the central zone and is composed of about 50 incompletely defined lobules with minute ducts that empty directly into the urethra just above the ejaculatory ducts.

The blood supply to the prostate gland is variable, most commonly arising from the common origin of the internal pudendal and inferior gluteal arteries off the internal iliac (hypogastric) arteries. The veins draining the prostate are wide and thin-walled, forming a plexus that communicates with the plexus draining the bladder into the internal iliac veins. The prostatic plexus also communicates with the vertebral venous plexuses; therefore, a tumor in the prostate may give rise to secondary growth in the vertebral column. Lymphatic drainage of the prostate follows that of the seminal vesicles and bladder neck into the iliac chain of nodes.

All the muscular tissue in the vas deferens, prostate, prostatic urethra and seminal vesicles is concerned with ejaculation. Prostate secretions contribute to the seminal fluid.

Penis

The penis is composed chiefly of cavernous (erectile) tissue and is traversed by the urethra. The posterior surface of the flaccid penis is

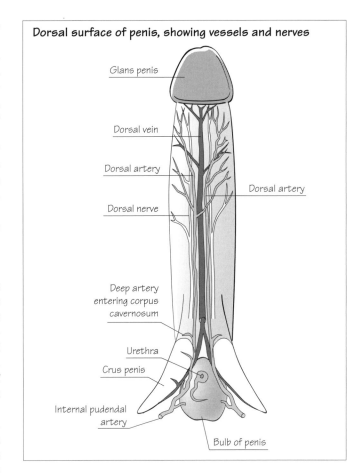

Dorsal surface of penis, showing vessels and nerves

Glans penis
Dorsal vein
Dorsal artery
Dorsal artery
Dorsal nerve
Deep artery entering corpus cavernosum
Urethra
Crus penis
Internal pudendal artery
Bulb of penis

nearest the urethra and the opposite, and more extensive surface, is dorsal. Most of the erectile tissue of the penis is arranged in three longitudinal columns, the paired **corpora cavernosa** and the single median **corpus spongiosum**. The cap of the penis, called the **glans**, is continuous with the spongiosum and also contains erectile tissue. Engorgement of the cavernous tissue with blood produces considerable enlargement of the penis and its erection. The glans of the penis is covered with a retractable folded layer of thin skin, called the prepuce or foreskin. It is this layer of skin that is removed by the operation of circumcision.

The blood supply to the penis is derived from the internal pudendal arteries that enter the organ on its dorsal surface and penetrate deep into the erectile tissue of the corpora cavernosa. The venous drainage enters the prostatic plexus either directly or through the dorsal vein of the penis. The lymphatic drainage of the penis is into the medial group of superficial inguinal lymph nodes. Innervation of the penis, which is critical for its erection, is derived from the pudendal nerve (2nd, 3rd, 4th sacral nerves) and from the pelvic autonomic plexuses.

The function of the penis is penetration and deposition of semen into the vagina of the female.

7 Microscopic anatomy of the male reproductive tract

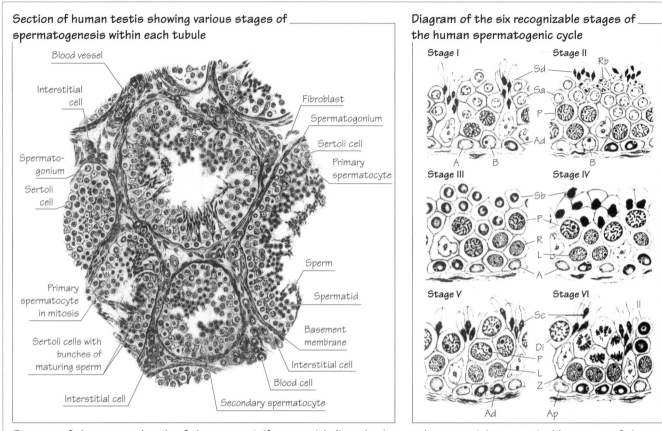

Section of human testis showing various stages of spermatogenesis within each tubule

- Blood vessel
- Interstitial cell
- Spermatogonium
- Sertoli cell
- Primary spermatocyte in mitosis
- Sertoli cells with bunches of maturing sperm
- Interstitial cell
- Fibroblast
- Spermatogonium
- Sertoli cell
- Primary spermatocyte
- Sperm
- Spermatid
- Basement membrane
- Interstitial cell
- Blood cell
- Secondary spermatocyte

Diagram of the six recognizable stages of the human spermatogenic cycle

Stage I, Stage II, Stage III, Stage IV, Stage V, Stage VI

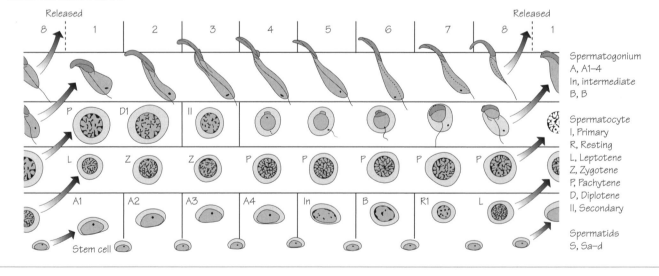

Diagram of the wave and cycle of the rat seminiferous epithelium. In the rat there are eight recognizable stages of the cycle: the four cell types consistently associated with each stage are identified in sequence as the entire course of one stem cell enters at A1

Spermatogonium
A, A1–4
In, intermediate
B, B

Spermatocyte
I, Primary
R, Resting
L, Leptotene
Z, Zygotene
P, Pachytene
D, Diplotene
II, Secondary

Spermatids
S, Sa–d

Testes

The testes have two distinct functions, spermatogenesis and androgen production. Spermatogenesis occurs within distinct structures called **seminiferous tubules** which lie coiled within lobules whose ducts all exit the testes into the epididymis centrally at the mediastinum. Androgen production occurs within pockets of specialized cells that lie in the interstitium between the tubules.

The cells responsible for spermatogenesis are arranged in distinct tubules surrounded by a basement membrane. The epithelium containing the developing spermatozoa that line the tubules is known as the **seminiferous epithelium**. In a cross-section of the testes, spermatocytes within a given tubule are in varying stages of maturation. Mixed among the spermatocytes are **Sertoli cells** that are the only non-germinal cells in the seminiferous epithelium. These cells, which were aptly called 'nurse cells' when first described by Sertoli in 1865, are responsible for the metabolic and structural support of the developing spermatozoa. The Sertoli cells all make contact with the basement membrane at one pole and surround the developing spermatozoa at the other. Sertoli cells have large, complex cytoplasmic 'fingers' which reach up and around many spermatozoa at one time.

Physiological studies have demonstrated that a wide variety of substances present in the circulation are excluded from the seminiferous tubule fluid, suggesting a **blood–testis barrier** similar to the blood–brain barrier. The ultrastructural basis of the blood–testis barrier is the tight junctions of the Sertoli cells that form between adjacent Sertoli cells. These cell barriers created by these tight junctions divide the germinal epithelium into basal and luminal compartments. The basement compartment contains the spermatogonia and the luminal compartment, the maturing germinal cells.

Spermatogenesis involves three phases: (i) mitotic proliferation to produce large numbers of cells; (ii) meiotic division to produce genetic diversity; and (iii) maturation which involves extensive cell modeling to facilitate the sperm reaching the oocyte in the female tract. Primitive spermatogonial stem cells that are activated at puberty are maintained in rounds of mitoses at the basement membrane of the seminiferous tubule. From this reservoir of self-regenerating stem cells emerge a morphologically distinct group of cells known as A spermatogonia. Each one of these A spermatogonia undergoes a limited number of mitotic divisions to form a 'clone' of germ cells. At the next to last mitotic division, the cells are known as B spermatogonia and, after the final division, as primary spermatocytes. The primary spermatocytes then undergo two meiotic cell divisions to halve the number of chromosomes in the daughter cells. Gonocytes undergoing the first of these meiotic divisions have very characteristic differences in their nuclear morphology that has led to a specific nomenclature (resting, leptotene, zygotene, pachytene and diplotene; Chapter 15). The first meiotic division produces secondary spermatocytes and the second, early haploid spermatids. The spermatids then undergo remarkable cytoplasmic re-modeling during which a tail, mitochondrial midpiece and acrosome all develop. Almost all the cytoplasm is expulsed except for a small droplet called the residual body that will be removed in the epididymis during the final maturation of the spermatozoon.

Development of the spermatozoa within the seminiferous epithelium is a complex and highly ordered sequence of events in most mammalian species. In humans, the process appears somewhat less orderly, but still follows the general principles found in other species. In each, the number of mitotic divisions the A1 spermatogonia undergo is fixed. In humans, four mitotic divisions occur. The length of time for an A1 spermatogonium to develop into a spermatozoon ready to enter the epididymis is also fixed and species specific. In humans, it takes 64 ± 4 days for this process. As the spermatocytes move through the maturation process, they also move in waves toward the lumen of the seminiferous tubule. These characteristics have been described as the 'spermatogenic cycle' and the 'wave of the seminiferous epithelium', respectively. The spermatogenic cycle is defined as the cellular associations that succeed one another cyclically in any given area of the seminiferous tubule. The waves of the seminiferous epithelium are the changes in the spatial relationships of the various cellular associations as one moves along the length of the tubule. In essence, the cycle represents in time what the wave represents in space.

The Sertoli cells in which the developing spermatozoa lie embedded are homologues of the granulosa cells in the ovary. Their functions include aromatization of androgen precursors to estrogen that has a local feedback on the androgen-producing (Leydig) cells and phagocytosis of the extruded spermatid cytoplasm. Sertoli cells also produce an androgen-binding protein.

The other function of the testes, androgen production, is performed by the **Leydig cells**. The Leydig cells are homologous with the theca cells of the ovary and produce large amounts of androgen from either circulating cholesterol or cholesterol made internally in the smooth endoplasmic reticulum. They are very large, foamy-appearing cells.

The most sensitive cells in the testis to damage are the spermatogonia. Irradiation, excessive alcohol intake, dietary deficiencies and local inflammation can induce degenerative changes. Excess heat induces extensive cell degeneration but does not affect the length of the spermatogenic cycle.

Epididymis and vas (ductus) deferens

The ducts forming the epididymis and vas deferens have muscular coats composed of an inner circular layer and an outer layer of longitudinally directed fibers. The muscle is responsible for peristalsis that moves the spermatozoa along the ducts. The ducts are lined with a mixture of secretory and ciliated cells.

Seminal vesicles

The alveoli of the seminal vesicles are lined with a pseudostratified epithelium whose cells contain numerous granules and clumps of yellow pigment. Some of the epithelial cells have flagella. The secretion of the seminal vesicles is a yellowish, viscous liquid containing globulin and fructose which provides the bulk of the ejaculate.

Prostate gland

The tubuloalveolar glands of the prostate are lined with an epithelium that is highly responsive to androgens. The acini of the central glandular zone that surrounds the ejaculatory ducts are large and irregular. By contrast, the acini of the peripheral glandular zone are small and regular. These striking differences in glandular architecture, along with the observation that several unique enzymes present in the seminal vesicles are present in the central but not the peripheral glandular zone, suggests different embryological tissue origins for these two parts of the prostate (Chapter 5.3). The epithelium of the prostatic tubuloalveolar glands is responsible for the acid phosphatase and citric acid normally found in semen.

Penis

The erectile tissue of the penis is a vast, spongelike system of irregular vascular spaces fed by the afferent arterioles and drained by the efferent venules. A pair of cylindrical bodies, the corpora cavernosa, are surrounded by a thick fibrous membrane called the tunica albuginea and separated by an incomplete fibrous septum. The veins draining the cavernous bodies lie just beneath the tunica. The interior of the cavernous bodies has many partitions called trabeculae within it. The trabeculae contain elastic fibers and smooth muscle embedded within thick bundles of collagen and are covered by endothelial cells.

8 Gross anatomy of the female reproductive tract

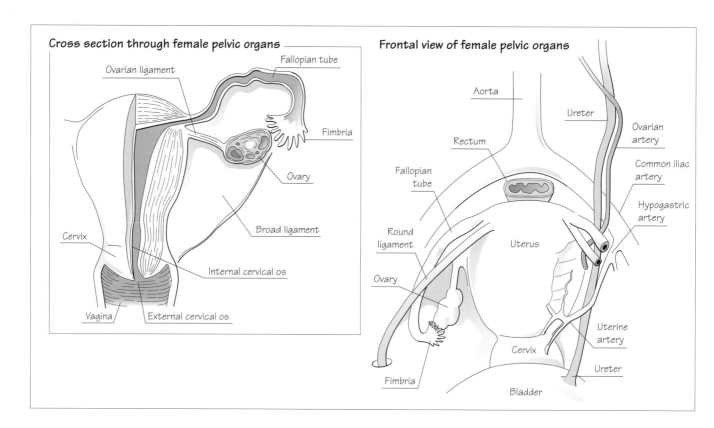

Cross section through female pelvic organs

Ovarian ligament
Fallopian tube
Fimbria
Ovary
Broad ligament
Internal cervical os
Cervix
Vagina
External cervical os

Frontal view of female pelvic organs

Aorta
Ureter
Ovarian artery
Rectum
Common iliac artery
Fallopian tube
Hypogastric artery
Round ligament
Uterus
Ovary
Uterine artery
Cervix
Ureter
Fimbria
Bladder

Ovaries

The ovaries are two small oval structures, $2 \times 4 \times 1.5$ cm, which lie deep in the female pelvis just lateral to, and behind, the uterus. They are loosely attached to the uterus by a connective tissue band. To the examiner performing a bimanual exam, they feel much like almonds sliding between the palpating fingers of the examiner's hand. After menopause, they may not even be palpable at all.

The blood supply to each ovary is the ovarian artery that arises from the aorta just below the renal artery and courses through the retroperitoneal space of the abdomen close to the ureter. The **venous drainage of the ovaries is into the vena cava on the right and the renal vein on the left**. This anatomic difference in venous drainage is important because the more lateral position of the left ovarian vein makes it more susceptible to obstruction and thrombus formation, especially in pregnancy. The lymphatic drainage of the ovary is into the lumbar (para-aortic) nodes.

The functions of the ovaries are to make large quantities of steroid hormones and to produce mature ova for fertilization.

Fallopian tubes

The Fallopian tubes are bilateral hollow structures that attach to the uterus at each cornua (corner). The Fallopian tube is divided anatomically and functionally into three sections, the **cornua**, **isthmus** and **fimbria**. The cornual section, which is contained within the muscular wall of the uterus, provides a stable, strong connection with the uterus. Fertilization occurs in the isthmus, which is the long, narrow pencil-

like portion of the tube. The fimbriated, or fluted end of the tube, is the most distal portion. The fimbria shows continual sweeping-like activity and can reach into the cul-de-sac to pick up ovulated eggs which fall behind the uterus.

The fimbria of the Fallopian tube is not enclosed within the parietal peritoneum of the broad ligament and hence communicates with the abdominal cavity. The opening of the tube directly into the abdominal cavity means that foreign matter that enters the vagina such as bacteria, sperm and chemicals can gain access to the abdominal cavity by traversing the cervical canal, uterus and Fallopian tube. This connection between the external environment and the female pelvis has important implications for intraperitoneal spread of infections ascending through the reproductive tract and for exposure to carcinogens (Chapters 42 and 39, respectively).

The blood supply to the Fallopian tube is largely through the ovarian vessels, although anastomoses with ascending branches of the uterine artery occur in the broad ligament. The lymph drainage of the tube follows the ovary into the para-aortic nodes.

The functions of the Fallopian tube are to transport sperm and eggs to the site of fertilization within the tube and to return the zygote to the uterine cavity for implantation.

Together with the Fallopian tubes, the ovaries are covered with a sheet of parietal peritoneum known as the **broad ligament**. The broad ligament forms a double-leaf filmy structure that is bounded superiorly by the round ligament of the uterus and connects the uterus, the Fallopian tubes and the ovaries to the pelvic sidewall just lateral to these structures. The broad ligament contains important blood vessels including the uterine artery and vein.

Uterus

The uterus is a single, pear-shaped, muscular structure that sits between the bladder and rectum in the female pelvis. A mature uterus weighs between 30 and 40 g in a woman who has never delivered a baby and 75–100 g in one who has. It is anchored in the pelvis by three sets of connective tissue ligaments: the **round, cardinal** and **uterosacral ligaments**. The round ligaments attach to the cornua just in front of the Fallopian tubes. These distinct cord-like structures traverse the pelvis, enter the inguinal rings bilaterally and attach firmly to the osteum of the pelvic bone. They provide stability for the upper pole of the uterus but are not essential for the organ's stability. The cardinal ligaments connect the uterus at the level of the cervix to the anterior abdominal wall. The uterosacral ligaments are attached to the uterus posteriorly at the level of the cervix and connect to the sacral bones. The cardinal and uterosacral ligaments provide significant support to the female pelvic floor. Damage to these ligaments, including undue stretching from childbirth, can cause prolapse of the uterus and pelvic floor down into the vagina or even through onto the vulva.

The uterus is divided into three anatomically and functionally distinct areas, the **cervix**, the **lower uterine segment** and the **corpus**. The cervix, which is composed largely of firm connective tissue, is about 4 cm in total length. About 2 cm of this length protrudes into the vagina and the remainder is intraperitoneal. The cervical opening into the uterus is the internal os and the opening into the vagina, the external os. The lower uterine segment is the lower third of the uterus and is composed largely of muscle. The lower segment draws the dilating cervix up and thins in labor. The corpus is the largest segment and is composed of thick muscle. The very top of the uterus between the Fallopian tubes is the fundus. The term **fundus** is sometimes used to refer to the entire corpus of the uterus.

The blood supply of the uterus is complex. The fundus is supplied by vessels stemming from the ovarian arteries while the corpus, lower segment and cervix are supplied by the uterine arteries. The uterine artery is the largest branch of the anterior division of the internal iliac artery (also known as the hypogastric artery). The uterine artery travels from the pelvic sidewall to the uterus at the level of the internal os of the cervix and the cardinal and uterosacral ligaments. In doing so, the uterine artery crosses over the ureter that is coursing directly from the kidney toward the bladder. This anatomical relationship must be kept in mind during all pelvic surgery that involves the uterus and its blood supply. Failure to remember that 'water runs under the bridge' has caused many an avoidable ureteral injury.

The lymphatic drainage of the uterus follows the blood supply. The fundus and upper part of the body drain to lymph nodes in the para-aortic chains whereas the lower part body of the uterus and the cervix drain into nodes located along the internal and external iliac vessels.

The function of the uterus is to provide support for the growing fetus during pregnancy.

Vagina

The vagina is a tubular structure that spans the distance between its opening at the introitus of the perineum and the cervix. Its surface is

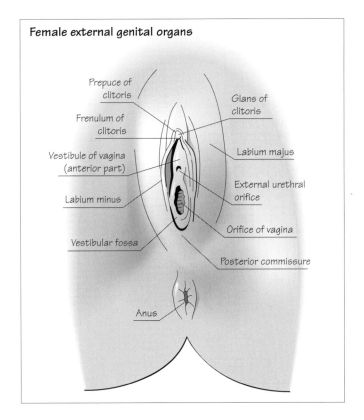

Female external genital organs

- Prepuce of clitoris
- Frenulum of clitoris
- Vestibule of vagina (anterior part)
- Labium minus
- Vestibular fossa
- Glans of clitoris
- Labium majus
- External urethral orifice
- Orifice of vagina
- Posterior commissure
- Anus

covered with a compliant, rugated-appearing epithelium. The upper two-thirds of the vagina is most correctly considered part of the internal genitalia because of its embryological relationship with the uterus. The hymen, which may remain as a thin transverse membrane through puberty or first sexual intercourse, is seen as an irregular circle of tissue at the opening of the vagina into the vulva.

The function of the vagina is to hold the male penis during intercourse and serve as a temporary receptacle for semen.

Vulva

The external female genitalia are collectively known as the vulva. The vulva comprises the **lower one-third of the vagina**, the **clitoris** and the **labia**. The labia majora are the largest structure and surround the other organs, ending in the mons pubis, which is a large fatty prominence that lies over the pelvic symphysis. The mons and the labia majora are the only visible parts of the female external genitalia. One must part the labia majora in order to see the labia minora, clitoris and urethral opening. There are **numerous mucus-secreting glands** lining the vaginal opening. The largest and most important of these are the Bartholin's glands which extend posterolaterally towards the buttocks.

The blood supply to the vulva is the internal pudendal artery that derives from the posterior division of the internal iliac artery. The lymph drainage is into the inguinal nodes.

The female clitoris is the homolog of the male penis and is the organ of sexual arousal in the female.

9 Microscopic anatomy of the female reproductive tract

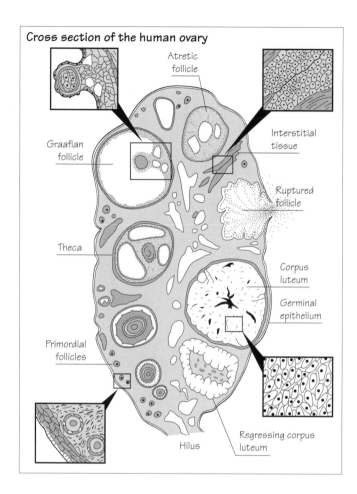

Cross section of the human ovary

- Atretic follicle
- Graafian follicle
- Interstitial tissue
- Ruptured follicle
- Theca
- Corpus luteum
- Germinal epithelium
- Primordial follicles
- Regressing corpus luteum
- Hilus

Ovary

The ovary has two distinct functions, germ cell production and steroid hormone biosynthesis. Germ cell support occurs in microscopic structures known as follicles. Unstimulated follicles each contain a primitive or **primordial oocyte** surrounded by a single layer of cells, the **granulosa cells**. Surrounding the granulosa cells are a collar of cells known as **theca cells**. Theca cells produce androgens that are then converted to estrogens by the granulosa cells (Chapter 3). Steroid hormones produced by the ovary act both within the follicle to support the developing oocyte and outside the ovary on target tissues.

The human ovary contains about 2 million oocytes at birth and about 100 000 at puberty. The number of oocytes continues to decrease throughout a woman's reproductive life span. This decrease occurs because mitosis of the primitive oogonia stops midway through fetal life and does not resume. At the time that mitosis stops, the newly formed oocytes enter into the prophase of the first meiotic division. They will remain in meiotic prophase until either they are stimulated to mature for ovulation or they shrivel and die, a process called **atresia**.

The primordial follicles are scattered just beneath the connective tissue capsule covering the ovary. This superficial position permits ovulation into the abdominal cavity. The earliest signs of follicular

growth are (i) an increase in size of the oocyte, (ii) a change in the shape of the granulosa cells from flat to cuboidal and an increase in their number and (iii) the appearance of a **zona pellucida** around the oocyte. The zona pellucida is a clear ring of gelatinous protein matrix immediately surrounding the oocyte. Once growth of the granulosa cells has produced three to four layers of cells, fluid begins to accumulate between the cells. This resembles blood plasma and contains high concentrations of several protein and steroid hormones. When the follicular fluid surrounds the oocyte, the follicle is known as a **Graafian follicle** and is approaching ovulation. Although as many as 20 follicles begin to mature in each wave of recruitment, typically only one successfully ovulates.

Ovulation involves expulsion of the egg through a thinned-out area known as the stigma. Stigmata can be seen with the naked eye as 'blisters' on the surface of the ovary. After the oocyte is released, the follicle collapses and the granulosa cells proliferate to fill the space. They undergo a remarkable transformation into plump, endocrinologically active cells known as lutein cells. The structure that forms is the **corpus luteum**, or yellow body, named for the yellow color of the pigment in the transformed cells. During corpus luteum formation, blood vessels penetrate the follicular basement membrane.

Fallopian tube

The Fallopian tube is covered by a columnar epithelium with long **cilia** on the surface of many of the cells. The cilia are constantly beating toward the uterus; their function is to facilitate movement of the non-motile zygote toward the uterine cavity for implantation. The importance of normal ciliary motion is demonstrated by pathologic implantation of an embryo (**ectopic pregnancy**) when the cilia have been injured.

Uterus

The uterus is composed largely of smooth muscle, the **myometrium**, and is lined with a glandular epithelium, the **endometrium**. Myometrial myocytes are smooth muscle cells attached by gap junctions, making them function as a large coordinated muscle mass. The uterus must be capable of enormous growth during pregnancy. This is accomplished by hypertrophy of the myocytes and by recruitment of new myocytes from stem cells within the myometrial connective tissue.

The endometrium is both an endocrine target organ and a gland. Under the influence of cyclic hormone production by the ovary, the endometrium undergoes striking microscopic changes in its glandular structure and function. During the preovulatory phase of the menstrual cycle, the epithelial cells on the surface of the endometrium proliferate profusely under the influence of estrogen. The glands proliferate and elongate deep into the subepithelial layer known as the endometrial stroma. Small muscular arteries known as **spiral arteries** grow upwards from the basal layer of the endometrium between the elongating glands. The hallmark of the **proliferative endometrium** is frequent mitoses in the epithelium. Immediately prior to ovulation, the glands are maximally elongated and markedly coiled.

With ovulation, the hormonal environment within the uterus changes from estrogen dominant to progesterone dominant. Mitosis ceases in the glandular epithelium and the cells form a single columnar layer within the glands. Within 2 days of ovulation, small subnuclear vacuoles form in the columnar cells. Rich in glycogen and lipid by 4 days after ovulation, these secretory vacuoles migrate to the luminal side of the cells. Over the next 2 days, the vacuoles discharge their contents into the glandular lumens leaving the borders of the glandular cells frayed in appearance. This activity is the basis for the term **secretory endometrium** used to describe the postovulatory changes.

Simultaneously with the glandular changes, the stromal cells enlarge and acquire a foamy appearance indicative of increased metabolism. These cells become very esosinophilic and are known as decidual cells. **Decidualization** of the endometrium begins around the elongated and coiled spiral arteries. Decidualization then spreads under the surface epithelium and glands by 10 days after ovulation.

If implantation does not occur, progesterone production by the corpus luteum stops by day 13–14 postovulation. The endometrium undergoes ischemic necrosis and sloughs off as menstruation. If pregnancy does occur, the extended life span of the corpus luteum will prolong the progesterone support and decidualization of the stroma will continue.

The stroma is an important source of several peptides in pregnancy, notably prolactin, insulin-like growth factor binding protein 1 (IGFBP-1) and parathyroid hormone-related peptide (PTHrP).

The changes in the endometrium are so predictable and hormone dependent that they can be used to document ovulation and its timing. Endometrial biopsies are typically taken in the postovulatory phase where the histological changes can be used to accurately date the interval from ovulation to within 1 day.

Cervix and vagina

The cervix is composed largely of connective tissue covered by a layer of mucus-secreting **glandular epithelium** inside the cervical canal and a **squamous epithelium** on the portion visible in the vagina. The transition between the glandular and squamous epithelium is known as the transformation zone. The **transformation zone** typically occurs just inside the external os of the cervix. The transformation zone is important in that it is a common site of dysplastic changes that can become malignant. The vagina is covered with squamous epithelium.

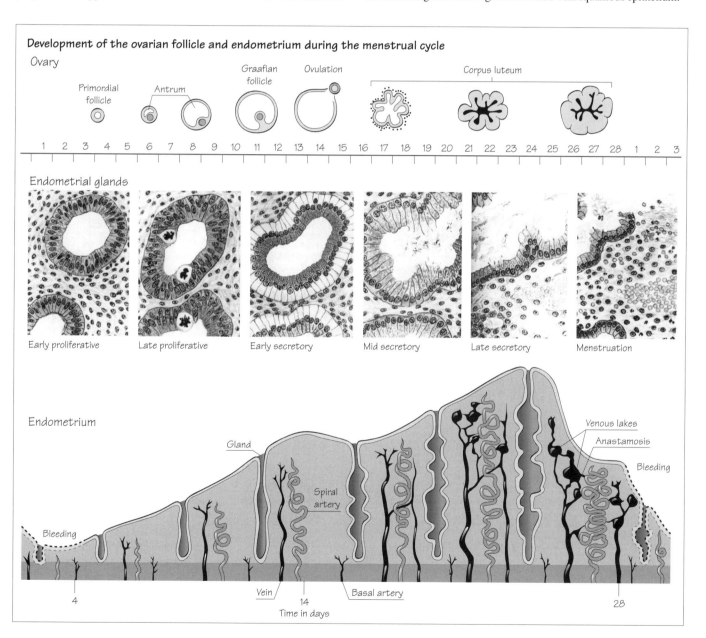

Development of the ovarian follicle and endometrium during the menstrual cycle

Ovary

Primordial follicle · Antrum · Graafian follicle · Ovulation · Corpus luteum

1 2 3 4 5 6 7 8 9 10 11 12 13 14 15 16 17 18 19 20 21 22 23 24 25 26 27 28 1 2 3

Endometrial glands

Early proliferative · Late proliferative · Early secretory · Mid secretory · Late secretory · Menstruation

Endometrium

Gland · Spiral artery · Venous lakes · Anastamosis · Bleeding · Bleeding · Vein · Basal artery

4 · 14 · 28

Time in days

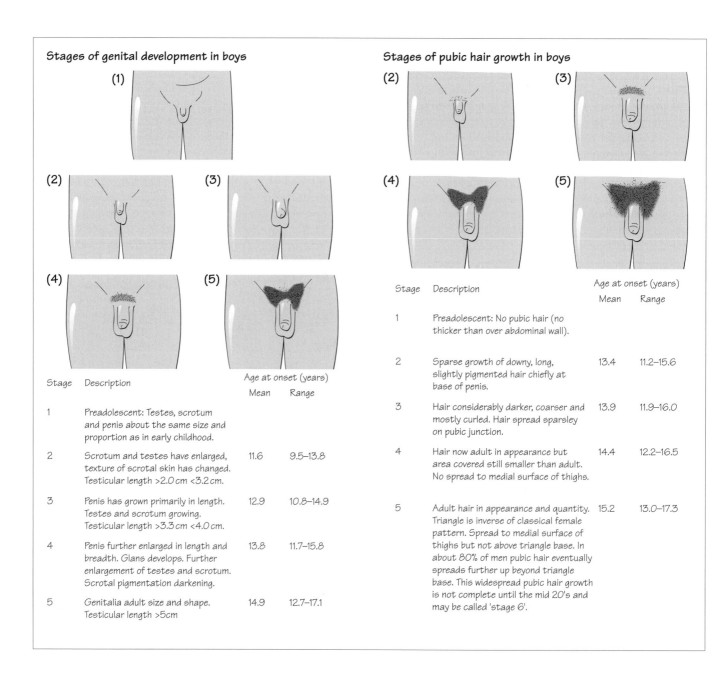

Stages of genital development in boys

(1)

(2)

(3)

(4)

(5)

Stage	Description	Age at onset (years)	
		Mean	Range
1	Preadolescent: Testes, scrotum and penis about the same size and proportion as in early childhood.		
2	Scrotum and testes have enlarged, texture of scrotal skin has changed. Testicular length >2.0 cm <3.2 cm.	11.6	9.5–13.8
3	Penis has grown primarily in length. Testes and scrotum growing. Testicular length >3.3 cm <4.0 cm.	12.9	10.8–14.9
4	Penis further enlarged in length and breadth. Glans develops. Further enlargement of testes and scrotum. Scrotal pigmentation darkening.	13.8	11.7–15.8
5	Genitalia adult size and shape. Testicular length >5cm	14.9	12.7–17.1

Stages of pubic hair growth in boys

(2)

(3)

(4)

(5)

Stage	Description	Age at onset (years)	
		Mean	Range
1	Preadolescent: No pubic hair (no thicker than over abdominal wall).		
2	Sparse growth of downy, long, slightly pigmented hair chiefly at base of penis.	13.4	11.2–15.6
3	Hair considerably darker, coarser and mostly curled. Hair spread sparsley on pubic junction.	13.9	11.9–16.0
4	Hair now adult in appearance but area covered still smaller than adult. No spread to medial surface of thighs.	14.4	12.2–16.5
5	Adult hair in appearance and quantity. Triangle is inverse of classical female pattern. Spread to medial surface of thighs but not above triangle base. In about 80% of men pubic hair eventually spreads further up beyond triangle base. This widespread pubic hair growth is not complete until the mid 20's and may be called 'stage 6'.	15.2	13.0–17.3

Puberty is the process by which the immature individual will acquire the physical and behavioral attributes which will allow him or her to reproduce. In males, it is largely the response of the body to widespread actions of androgens secreted by the newly awakened testes, under the influence of gonadotropins secreted by the anterior pituitary.

Physical changes of puberty

In North America and Europe, puberty in boys visibly begins between ages 9 and 14 years with enlargement of the testes. Secondary sexual characteristics will progressively appear over the ensuing 2–2.5 years.

Facial hair, which is the last secondary sexual characteristic to appear, will not be fully mature until age 20–25 years.

The physical changes of puberty in boys have been divided into five stages using a descriptive system developed by Marshall and Tanner. These investigators examined groups of English boys as they went through sexual maturation and classified the relative and absolute changes in their sexual characteristics. Although they did not regard their findings as universal, the classification system they derived has been widely used to describe and show these changes.

Adrenarche

Adrenarche is the contribution of the adrenal gland to puberty. It is characterized by an increase in adrenal synthesis and secretion of the weak androgens: androstenedione, dehydroepiandrosterone (DHEA), and dehydroepiandrosterone sulfate (DHEA-S). Although the adrenal gland contributes only 5% of the total circulating androgen pool in boys, these adrenal androgens are responsible for initiating axillary and pubic hair growth. They are converted in the periphery to the more potent androgens: testosterone and dihydrotestosterone (DHT). Testosterone and DHT then stimulate pubic and axillary hair growth as well as axillary sebaceous glands. The appearance of axillary and pubic hair occurs in parallel with increasing testicular size and visibly marks the onset of puberty.

The exact trigger for adrenarche is not known. The best evidence is that it is an intrinsic, programmed event within the adrenal gland that is independent of adrenocorticotropic hormone (ACTH).

Testicular maturation

Maturation of the testes at puberty involves initiation of androgen production by the Leydig cells, growth of the seminiferous tubules and initiation of spermatogenesis. All three of these events are controlled by the gonadotropins: follicle-stimulating hormone (FSH) and luteinizing hormone (LH).

Throughout childhood, FSH and LH concentrations in both the pituitary and plasma are low. Pulse amplitude and frequency of both hormones are also low, suggesting that the gonadotropin-releasing hormone (GnRH) pulse generator is cycling slowly (juvenile pause). About a year before testicular enlargement appears, the release of pulsatile FSH and LH begins to increase in both amplitude and concentration, most notably during sleep. This marked diurnal rhythm in FSH and LH secretion is the first endocrinological manifestation of puberty. Diurnal variations are notable during puberty, but are almost obliterated by the end of puberty.

The initiation of puberty is thought to occur via the release of central nervous system inhibition of the hypothalamic GnRH pulse generator. The site and exact mechanism of inhibitory release are not known; however, most evidence indicates that the trigger also resides in the CNS. Individuals who lack the hypothalamic GnRH pulse generator do not undergo puberty (Kallman syndrome, see Chapter 27), and tumors or surgery in the region of the median basal hypothalamus are associated with delayed or absent puberty.

The increase in size of the testes is largely the result of increasing mass of the seminiferous tubules and initiation of spermatogenesis. Leydig cell stimulation, which results in a tenfold increase in testosterone production over the course of puberty, accounts for only a small proportion of the change in testicular size, because the Leydig cells occupy less than 10% of the total testicular mass.

Secondary sexual characteristics

Testosterone and its metabolites cause the following somatic changes in pubertal boys:
- Increased laryngeal size.
- Deepening of the voice.
- Increased bone mass.
- Increased mass and strength of skeletal muscle.
- Thickened skin.
- Increased and thickened hair on the trunk, pubis, axillae and face.

Somatic growth

Somatic growth at puberty is the result of a complex interaction between gonadal sex steroids, growth hormone (GH) and insulin-like growth factor I (IGF-I). Insulin and thyroxine are also necessary for optimal growth. The absence of either GH, IGF-I or IGF-I receptor will lead to somatic dwarfism, even in the presence of normal plasma sex steroid concentrations.

Concomitant with the changes in pulse frequency of LH that signal the beginning of puberty is a change in amplitude of GH secretion. This change appears to be the result of estrogen stimulation in both boys and girls. In boys, while the increase in GH can be initiated and maintained by testosterone, it does not occur with the administration of DHT, and GH secretion in the presence of testosterone can be blocked by the administration of tamoxifen, an estrogen receptor blocker. By contrast, even miniscule doses of estrogen substantially increase GH concentrations. These findings suggest that the effect of testosterone on bone growth is indirect and probably secondary to aromatization of testosterone to estradiol. This contrasts with testosterone action on muscle, where androgens act directly to increase muscle mass.

Bone growth occurs when testosterone, aromatized to estradiol, increases GH levels, thus causing a parallel rise in IGF-I. IGF-I is a potent anabolic hormone that mediates many metabolic actions of GH, including trabecular bone formation. Under normal circumstances GH stimulates IGF-I synthesis, and IGF-I suppresses GH release in a negative feedback loop. At puberty, however, GH continues to rise despite high levels of circulating IGF-I, allowing for maximum linear growth. Outside of puberty, this combination of an increase in both GH and IGF-I is seen only in acromegaly, where GH secretion is autonomous. Peak growth velocity in boys occurs when plasma testosterone levels reach 50% of adult male levels, and growth will continue until epiphyseal fusion occurs in the long bones. The sex steroids (perhaps via estrogen activity) are responsible for epiphyseal closure, which occurs at a median of 21 years of age in boys.

The determinants of final adult height are many and include genetic predisposition, body mass index at the onset of puberty, nutrition and length of puberty. Genetic determinants of bone growth appear to be carried on the distal short arm of the X chromosome. This locus does not appear to undergo X inactivation and hence it, and any homologous loci on the Y chromosome, will contribute to final adult height. This is particularly notable in men with the sex chromosome disorder Klinefelter syndrome (XXY). Men with Klinefelter syndrome are unusually tall, presumably because of the double dose of the X-linked stature determinants.

Higher body mass indices in late childhood affect ultimate height because both boys and girls who have increased body fat tend to enter puberty earlier. They begin their growth spurt after a shorter period of prepubertal growth and hence may not grow as tall as genetically predispositioned. A longer period of prepubertal growth is also one of the two reasons why men tend to be taller than women; the other is that boys achieve a greater peak linear growth velocity during adolescence than girls.

Androgens have a direct anabolic effect on muscle mass to increase it during puberty.

11 Puberty in girls

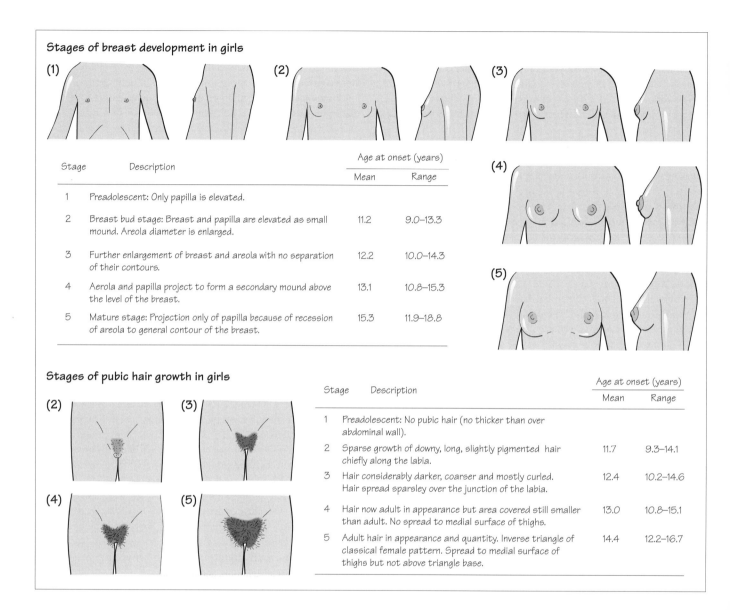

Stages of breast development in girls

Stage	Description	Age at onset (years)	
		Mean	Range
1	Preadolescent: Only papilla is elevated.		
2	Breast bud stage: Breast and papilla are elevated as small mound. Areola diameter is enlarged.	11.2	9.0–13.3
3	Further enlargement of breast and areola with no separation of their contours.	12.2	10.0–14.3
4	Aerola and papilla project to form a secondary mound above the level of the breast.	13.1	10.8–15.3
5	Mature stage: Projection only of papilla because of recession of areola to general contour of the breast.	15.3	11.9–18.8

Stages of pubic hair growth in girls

Stage	Description	Age at onset (years)	
		Mean	Range
1	Preadolescent: No pubic hair (no thicker than over abdominal wall).		
2	Sparse growth of downy, long, slightly pigmented hair chiefly along the labia.	11.7	9.3–14.1
3	Hair considerably darker, coarser and mostly curled. Hair spread sparsley over the junction of the labia.	12.4	10.2–14.6
4	Hair now adult in appearance but area covered still smaller than adult. No spread to medial surface of thighs.	13.0	10.8–15.1
5	Adult hair in appearance and quantity. Inverse triangle of classical female pattern. Spread to medial surface of thighs but not above triangle base.	14.4	12.2–16.7

As mentioned in Chapter 10, puberty is the process by which the immature individual will acquire the physical and behavioral attributes which will allow him or her to reproduce. In girls, it is largely the response of the body to widespread actions of estrogens secreted by the newly awakened ovary, under the influence of gonadotropins secreted by the anterior pituitary.

Physical changes of puberty

In North American and European girls, puberty visibly begins between ages 8 and 10 with breast development. Other secondary sexual characteristics will appear over the ensuing 2.5 years. Puberty culminates in girls with the onset of menstruation. The average age of menarche in Caucasian girls is 12.8 ± 1.2 (S.D.) years. Menarche occurs an average of 4 months earlier in African-American girls.

The physical changes of puberty in girls have been divided into five stages using a descriptive system developed by Marshall and Tanner. These investigators examined groups of English girls as they went through sexual maturation and classified the relative and absolute changes in their sexual characteristics. Although they did not regard their findings as universal, the classification system they derived has been widely used to describe and show these changes.

Adrenarche

Adrenarche is the contribution of the adrenal gland to puberty in both girls and boys. It is a developmentally programmed increase in adrenal synthesis and secretion of the weak androgens: androstenedione, dehydroepiandrosterone (DHEA) and dehydroepiandrosterone sulfate (DHEA-S). Adrenarche begins at about age 6–8 years in girls. The secretion of these weak adrenal androgens precedes the visible onset of puberty by about 2 years. DHEA and DHEA-S are responsible for initiating the growth of pubic and axillary hair as well as axillary sebaceous glands. The appearance of axillary and pubic hair occurs in parallel with the beginning of breast development and visibly marks the onset of puberty in girls.

The exact trigger for adrenarche is not known. It is independent of ACTH release, gonadotropin release, and ovarian function, and appears to be an intrinsic, programmed event within the adrenal gland.

Menarche

Menarche is the term used to describe the onset of menstrual cycles in girls. It is the culmination of a complex sequence of events that involves maturation of the hypothalamic–pituitary–ovarian axis to produce mature ova and an endometrium that can support a zygote if fertilization should occur. The three stages of maturation include (i) increased release of follicle-stimulating hormone (FSH) and luteinizing hormone (LH) from the pituitary, (ii) ovarian response to gonadotropins to produce steroids and (iii) establishment of positive feedback to estrogens which permits ovulation to begin.

Throughout childhood, FSH and LH concentrations in the pituitary and plasma of boys and girls are low. As described in Chapter 10, the pulse amplitude and frequency of FSH and LH are also low, suggesting the gonadotropin-releasing hormone (GnRH) pulse generator is cycling slowly (juvenile pause). The first endocrinological manifestation of puberty is an increase in FSH and LH pulsation amplitude during sleep. Puberty appears to be initiated by release of central nervous system inhibition of the hypothalamic GnRH pulse generator. The diurnal sleep–awake difference in FSH and LH secretion is almost obliterated by the end of puberty.

There has been much interest in the observation that the age of menarche decreased by 2–3 months per decade during the 150 years preceding World War II and then stabilized over the following 50 years. This decrease is thought to represent the influence of optimal nutrition. The onset of menarche is closely related to the attainment of a crucial percentage of body fat. Recently two metabolic signals have been identified which can act centrally: insulin-like growth factor I (IGF-I) and leptin. Serum IGF-I levels increase during childhood and peak at puberty: the increase parallels that of DHEA-S, the marker of adrenarche. Leptin, a hormone signaling satiety, inhibits neuropeptide Y (NPY). NPY is a mediator of food intake and GnRH neuronal activity in the hypothalamus. **Rising leptin levels inhibit NPY, thereby releasing GnRH from its prepubertal inhibition.**

Maturation of the ovary at puberty involves initiation of estrogen production by the granulosa cells surrounding the ova. Waves of granulosa cells undergo development and then atresia as puberty progresses. Ova begin to mature under the influence of ovarian estrogen produced by the granulosa cells, culminating in ovulation. With ovulation of the first ovum, progesterone production by the corpus luteum begins. The endometrium responds to the estrogen by proliferating and to the progesterone by converting to a secretory stage capable of supporting implantation. Initially, when girls reach menarche, some of their cycles are anovulatory because of incomplete maturation of the hypothalamic

positive feedback response to estrogen. The bleeding that occurs represents continuous exposure of the endometrium to estrogen and is really sloughing of proliferative or hyperplastic endometrium. This type of bleeding is very unpredictable and can be quite heavy because the tissue lacks the progesterone effect that makes menstruation a self-limited phenomenon. By 5 years after the onset of menarche, 90% of girls have regular, ovulatory cycles.

Breast development (thelarche)

The mammary gland, or breast, is an ectodermal derivative that is very hormone sensitive both embryologically and after puberty. The basic pattern of breast structure is common to all mammals in spite of wide variations in the number of mammary glands and their size, location and shape. Each mammary gland is a lobulated mass of glandular tissue, fibrous tissue that connects the lobes, and adipose tissue between the lobes. Each of the lobes contains lobules of alveoli, blood vessels and lactiferous ducts. A more detailed description of the structure and function of the human breast may be found in Chapter 20.

At birth, the breasts consist almost entirely of lactiferous ducts with few, if any, alveoli. These rudimentary mammary glands are capable of a small degree of secretory function (witch's milk) within a few days of birth. This secretion occurs because of the high prolactin levels in the newborn infant and the exposure of the fetal breast to high concentrations of placental estrogen during gestation. Once the placental estrogen is cleared from the neonatal circulation, the breast enters a quiescent phase until puberty.

With the onset of puberty, ovarian estrogens induce growth of the lactiferous duct system. The ducts themselves branch and grow and their ends begin to form into small solid spheroidal masses of cells that will later become lobular alveoli. The breast enlarges, as does the areola. Subsequent to the establishment of cyclic estrogen and progesterone secretion following menarche, additional ductal and rudimentary lobular growth will occur. The breasts will continue to increase somewhat in size due to deposition of fat and additional connective tissue. Adrenal corticosteroids further enhance duct development. Final differentiation and growth of the breast will not occur until pregnancy.

Secondary sexual characteristics

Ovarian estrogens also produce the following changes in pubertal girls:
• Pubic hair.
• Keratinization (cornification) of the vaginal mucosa.
• Enlargement of labia minora and majora.
• Uterine enlargement.
• Increased fat deposition in hips and thighs.

Somatic growth

The pubertal growth spurt in girls typically begins 2 years before it begins in boys. This difference accounts for about 50% of the 12 cm difference in average height between men and women. The other 50% is due to a slower rate of growth during the spurt in girls compared with boys. The mechanism by which sex steroids induce bone growth in girls is the same as in boys (Chapter 10). Structural growth ceases at a median age of 17 years in girls.

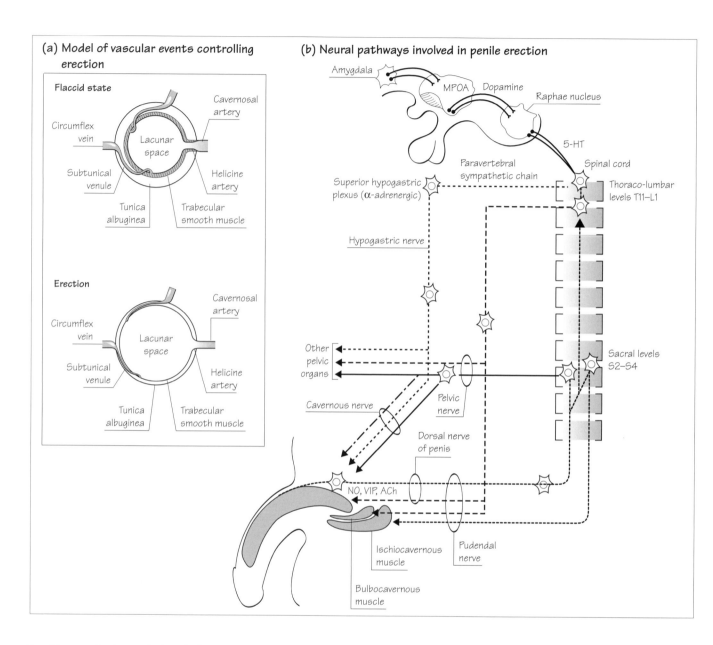

(a) Model of vascular events controlling erection

Flaccid state

Circumflex vein
Cavernosal artery
Lacunar space
Subtunical venule
Helicine artery
Tunica albuginea
Trabecular smooth muscle

Erection

Circumflex vein
Cavernosal artery
Lacunar space
Subtunical venule
Helicine artery
Tunica albuginea
Trabecular smooth muscle

(b) Neural pathways involved in penile erection

Amygdala
MPOA
Dopamine
Raphae nucleus
5-HT
Spinal cord
Paravertebral sympathetic chain
Thoraco-lumbar levels T11–L1
Superior hypogastric plexus (α-adrenergic)
Hypogastric nerve
Other pelvic organs
Sacral levels S2–S4
Cavernous nerve
Pelvic nerve
Dorsal nerve of penis
NO, VIP, ACh
Ischiocavernous muscle
Pudendal nerve
Bulbocavernous muscle

Erection, emission and ejaculation

An erection is a complex neuropsychological event that occurs when blood rapidly flows into the penis and becomes trapped in its spongy chambers. The three systems directly involved in a penile erection are (i) the spongy corpora cavernosa, (ii) the autonomic innervation and (iii) the blood supply of the penis. Sensory, peripheral and central nervous system pathways integrate the response within context.

Although there are three erectile bodies within the penis, the two corpora cavernosa are primarily responsible for penile rigidity during an erection. The corpus spongiosum becomes tumescent during an erection, but does not become rigid. It serves to redistribute the intraurethral pressure so that the urethra remains patent and an effective conduit for the ejaculate.

The basic physiology of an erection is best understood if one considers each corpus cavernosum as if it were a single lacunar chamber (see part (a) of figure above). Small (helicine) arteries drain into the lacunar space, which is bounded by smooth muscle within the trabecular wall. Exiting from the lacunar space are small venules that coalesce into larger (subtunical) venules. The subtunical venules drain through the tunica albuginea and form the emissary veins.

When the penis is flaccid, the smooth muscle in the lacunar walls is in a contracted state. This contracted state is maintained by noradrenergic sympathetic fibers. With activation of the parasympathetic system, the noradrenergic tone is blocked and the intralacunar smooth muscle relaxes. Blood flows easily into the lacunar space through the helicine arteries. The subtunical venules and the emissary veins are physically compressed by the expanded lacunae. In essence, the lacunar space becomes a large vascular 'sink' into which blood rapidly flows and becomes trapped when the intralacunar pressure equals the mean arterial pressure.

Regulation of cavernosal smooth muscle is thus central to control of an erection. Filling of the sinusoidal spaces with blood due to smooth muscle relaxation results from parasympathetic neural pathway activation and simultaneous inhibition of sympathetic outflow. The parasympathetic outflow travels to the penis through the pelvic nerve whereas the sympathetic outflow travels in the hypogastric nerve. Numerous neurotransmitters are involved in the parasympathetic modulation of cavernosal smooth muscle relaxation while contraction appears largely to be under α-noradrenergic control. Nitric oxide, which colocalizes with acetylcholine and vasoactive intestinal peptide (VIP) in nerve fibers terminating in the trabeculae of the corpora cavernosa and on the helicine arteries, is the primary pro-erectile neurotransmitter. Norepinephrine is the major anti-erectile agent.

Reflex erection can be elicited by afferent signals from sensory nerve endings on the glans; this reflex is mediated at the level of the spinal cord. The afferent limb of the reflex is carried by the internal pudendal nerves, which can also be activated by tactile stimulation of the perineum near the testes and scrotum. Erections can be modulated by supraspinal influences in the central nervous system. Serotonergic pathways within the raphe nucleus of the midbrain can inhibit erections. The hypothalamic medial preoptic area appears to be an important higher integrating center as is the amygdala. Dopamine is the candidate neurotransmitter in erectile control at this level.

The importance of testosterone in erectile function is not known. Nocturnal erections, which occur during episodes of rapid eye movement sleep, are testosterone dependent, whereas erections that occur in response to visual stimuli are not, and will occur in hypogonadal men.

As ejaculation approaches, penile turgor further increases and the smooth muscles in the prostate, vas deferens and seminal vesicles contract sequentially to expel the seminal plasma and spermatozoa into the urethra. This process, which is known as emission, is mediated by α-adrenergic sympathetic fibers in the hypogastric nerve. Ejaculation, which is the ejection of semen from the posterior urethra, occurs when the smooth muscles of the urethra and the striated bulbocavernosis and ischiocavernosis muscles contract.

Hormonal control of spermatogenesis

Ongoing spermatogenesis in the testes can be maintained qualitatively by testosterone alone; however, follicle-stimulating hormone (FSH) is required for initiation of spermatogenesis. The primary site of action of FSH within the seminiferous epithelium is in the Sertoli cells. FSH, delivered to the interstitial area of the testis via the small arterioles, diffuses through the basement membrane of the seminiferous tubules and binds to specific plasma membrane receptors on the Sertoli cells. Activation of the FSH receptors results in the synthesis of both intracellular androgen receptor and an androgen-binding protein (ABP). ABP is then secreted from the Sertoli cells where it binds androgens produced by the Leydig cells that have diffused from their interstitial site of production into the seminiferous tubule. ABP transfers the androgens to the germ cells where the androgens will be retained in promeiotic cells that contain androgen receptors. Although it is likely that nuclear receptor–gene interactions occur in the target germinal elements, their exact nature is not known. Once FSH initiates spermatogenesis, it will proceed as long as an adequate and uninterrupted supply of testosterone is available.

The FSH dependence of the Sertoli cells is analogous to the FSH control of their homologs in the ovary, the granulosa cells. In addition to ABP, the Sertoli cells secrete inhibin and activin as do follicular phase ovarian granulosa cells. Inhibin, along with testosterone, inhibits pituitary FSH secretion in the male. Activin receptors have been identified on spermatogenic cells and may be involved in FSH initiation of spermatogenesis.

Leydig cell function

Like the homologous theca cells in the ovary, Leydig cells respond to LH by synthesizing and secreting testosterone in a dose-dependent manner. In addition to LH receptors, receptors for prolactin and inhibin are found on Leydig cells. Both prolactin and inhibin facilitate the stimulatory activity of LH on testosterone production but neither stimulates it alone.

Regulation of gonadotropin secretion in males

The neuroendocrine mechanisms that regulate testicular function are fundamentally similar to those that regulate ovarian function. Hypothalamic GnRH, secreted in a pulsatile fashion into the portal system, acts on the pituitary of the male to release the gonadotropins, FSH and LH. These two gonadotropins, in turn, regulate the spermatogenic and endocrine activities of the testis. The same negative feedback mechanisms that inhibit gonadotropin release by the pituitary are operative in the male and female. The major difference between regulation of the male and female gonad is that gametogenesis and testosterone production occur continuously in the postpubertal male and not cyclically as in the female. The lack of cyclicity in males occurs because androgens do not exert a positive feedback on gonadotropin release.

Testosterone is the major regulator of LH secretion in the male. The negative feedback effect of testosterone is achieved largely by decreasing the frequency of the GnRH pulses released by the hypothalamus. There is also some reduction in GnRH pulse amplitude. Testosterone also inhibits FSH release but its effects are not as pronounced as they are on LH. The combination of the Sertoli cell hormone, inhibin (Chapter 2), and testosterone produces maximal FSH suppression.

13 The menstrual cycle

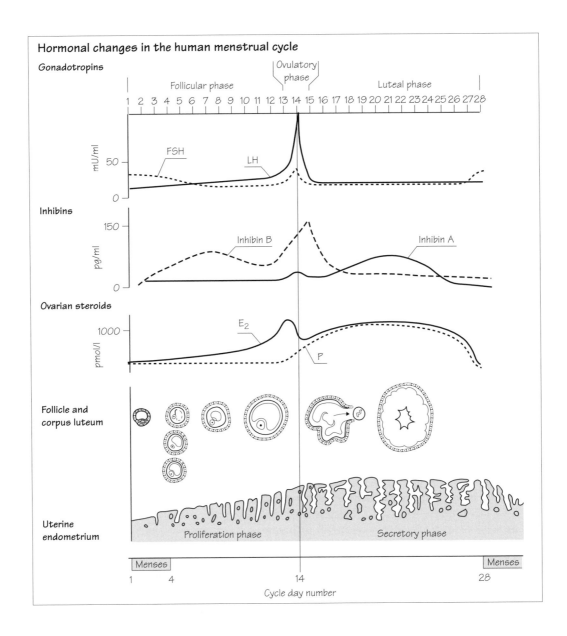

Hormonal changes in the human menstrual cycle

Unlike the mature male, in which gametogenesis and steroidogenesis proceed in a continuous fashion, the postpubertal human female exhibits repetitive cyclic changes in the hypothalamic–pituitary–ovarian axis which produce both gametes and a uterine environment prepared to support a pregnancy should fertilization occur. In the absence of conception, each cycle ends in menstrual bleeding. The pituitary gonadotropins, luteinizing hormone (LH) and follicle-stimulating hormone (FSH), are the links between the hypothalamus and the ovary that produce the cyclic changes.

The human menstrual cycle is best understood if divided into four phases based on functional and morphological changes in the ovary. These phases are (i) follicular, (ii) ovulatory, (iii) luteal and (iv) menstrual.

Follicular phase

The phase of the menstrual cycle leading up to ovulation is called the follicular phase. Although the follicular phase typically occupies the first half of the cycle, its length can vary. In ovulatory cycles of more or less than 28 days' duration, the deviation from the average is largely due to differences in the length of the follicular phase.

The follicular phase of the cycle is characterized by a progressive increase in the synthesis and release of **estradiol** and **inhibin B** from the **developing Graffian follicle** into both the follicular fluid and the systemic circulation. Progression of the follicle from its primordial or resting state in the ovary begins about 2 days before the onset of menstruation. At that time, the death of the corpus luteum from the previous cycle and the resultant rapid decline in estradiol, and to a lesser degree, progesterone and inhibin A, release the central inhibition of FSH secretion. In addition, the pulse frequency of LH begins to increase.

During the first 4–5 days of the follicular phase, recruitment or development of the early ovarian follicles continues. FSH induces granulosa cell proliferation and aromatase activity thereby increasing the amount of estradiol produced from thecal androgens. The recruited follicles now have several layers of granulosa cells surrounding their oocytes and a small accumulation of follicular fluid. In addition, FSH induces synthesis of additional FSH receptors as well as new LH receptors on the granulosa cells, thereby initiating LH responsiveness.

By days 5–7 of the cycle, a single follicle predominates which will mature and ovulate between days 13 and 15. The predominant follicle is characterized by the highest mitotic index of all the recruited follicles, by an optimal capacity for FSH retention in the follicular fluid and by high estradiol and inhibin B synthesis. Non-dominant follicles have an elevated androgen : estrogen ratio in their follicular fluid, suggesting suboptimal induction of aromatase. These non-dominant follicles will undergo **atresia**. The androgens may be key to the process of atresia itself, as granulosa cells treated with androgen *in vitro* undergo apoptosis.

During the mid- to late follicular phase, the rising estradiol and inhibin B levels in the circulation suppress FSH secretion, thereby preventing new follicular recruitment. The rising estradiol also leads to more LH secretion by the pituitary as well as increased ovarian responsiveness to the gonadotropin. Lastly, high estrogen levels cause growth of the endometrial tissue lining the uterus. These visible changes in the endometrium are defined as the 'proliferative phase' (Chapter 9).

Ovulatory phase

The ovulatory phase is characterized by a surge in pituitary LH secretion, which culminates in extrusion of the mature ovum through the capsule of the ovary. During the 2–3 days preceding the onset of the LH surge, circulating estradiol and inhibin B rise rapidly and in parallel. Estradiol synthesis is at a maximum and no longer FSH dependent. Progesterone begins to rise as the surging LH induces progesterone synthesis by the granulosa cells.

Key to ovulation is the midcycle positive feedback effect of estrogen on LH secretion. Proof that rising ovarian estrogens are central to ovulation lies in the observations that a gonadotropin surge can be elicited when rising circulating estradiol concentrations are produced experimentally by exogenous estrogen administration for 2–3 days in women and other primates. Progesterone made by the ovary augments the effects of estrogen, further indicating that the ovary, not the hypothalamus, is the site of the ovulatory 'clock' in primates.

The site of the positive feedback actions of midcycle estrogen appears to be in both the hypothalamic neuroendocrine cells and the pituitary gonadotropes. The exact site and mechanism by which estrogen induces the midcycle LH surge is unknown, but it appears to involve dopaminergic and β-endorphinergic neuronal modulation of the GnRH pulse generator to produce a 20-fold increase in sensitivity of the pituitary gonadotropes to GnRH. The GnRH pulse generator can be inhibited by both synthetic and naturally occuring opioids, suggesting that opioids play a pivotal role in the neuronal control of the midcycle LH surge. A small rise in FSH occurs simultaneously with the pronounced rise in LH at midcycle, presumably in response to the GnRH signal.

The mechanism by which ovulation occurs is not exactly clear but appears to require LH. Because LH has been shown to stimulate prostaglandin biosynthesis by ovarian cells and because inhibitors of prostaglandin synthesis inhibit ovulation in animals, prostaglandins are

hypothesized to be at least one of the mediators. Plasminogen activator, a serine protease that converts plasminogen to the proteolytically active enzyme plasmin, is produced by ovarian cells in response to FSH and may be involved in ovulation as well.

Luteal phase

After ovulation, the formation and maintenance of the corpus luteum and its production of progesterone becomes the dominant functional feature. In humans, the luteal cells make large amounts of estrogen and inhibin as well as progesterone and 17-hydroxyprogestrone, all of which are found in the systemic circulation. Although the estrogen concentrations are in the preovulatory positive feedback range, the uniquely high concentrations of progesterone prevent the estrogen from stimulating another LH surge from the pituitary. Instead, in the presence of these high concentrations of progesterone and estrogen, the preovulatory GnRH pulses are reduced in frequency, resulting in only baseline FSH and LH secretion.

The length of the luteal phase is normally 14 ± 2 days. If pregnancy does not ensue, the corpus luteum spontaneously regresses and follicular development proceeds for the next cycle. Small amounts of LH are necessary to maintain the corpus luteum in a normal cycle; however, after 14 days basal LH secretion will no longer support the endocrine function of the gland. The exact trigger for the demise of the corpus luteum is not known but the DNA fragmentation pattern of apoptosis appears in mid- and late luteal cells. If pregnancy ensues, maintenance of the corpus luteum and its progesterone production is critical to the success of the early gestation. Chorionic gonadotropin (hCG), a homologous hormone to LH secreted by gestational trophoblast, maintains the corpus luteum until the trophoblast assumes the role of progesterone secretion in pregnancy (Chapter 17). High levels of progesterone also create the 'secretory phase' of the endometrium. This phase is marked by endometrial maturation so that implantation can occur (Chapter 9).

The rise in FSH secretion that occurs near the end of the luteal phase is dependent on a concomitant drop in the high circulating levels of progesterone, estradiol and inhibin. Of clinical significance is the finding that an estrogen antagonist such as clomiphene citrate, administered in the luteal phase, causes a rise in circulating FSH levels and initiation of follicular recruitment.

Menstrual phase

The first day of menstruation actually marks the beginning of the next cycle. A new wave of follicles has been recruited and is progressing toward the Graffian stage. The phenomenon known as menstruation is largely an endometrial event that is triggered by the loss of progesterone support from the corpus luteum.

The biochemical basis for the dramatic structural changes that occur in the endometrium during menstruation are only partially understood. Specific hormonally regulated matrix-degrading proteases and lysosomes appear to be involved. The matrix-degrading proteases are part of the metalloproteinase (MMP) family of enzymes whose substrates include collagen and other matrix proteins. Of the MMP family, seven members are expressed in cell- and menstrual cycle-specific patterns. In addition, the endothelins, which are potent vasoconstrictors, appear to have maximum activity at the end of the luteal phase. Finally, the premenstrual fall in progesterone is associated with a decline in 15-hydroxyprostaglandin dehydrogenase activity, which increases the availability of prostaglandin $PGF_{2\alpha}$, a potent stimulator of myometrial contractility.

14 Human sexual response

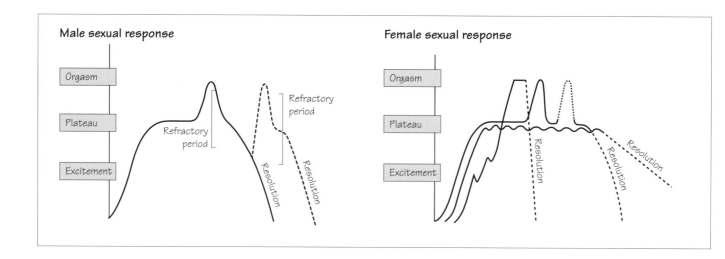

In view of the pervicacious gonadal urge in human beings, it is not a little curious that science develops its sole timidity about the pivotal point of the physiology of sex. Perhaps this avoidance … not of the bizarre and the extreme, the abnormal and the diseased, but of the normal usages and medial standards of mankind … perhaps this shyness is begotten by the certainty that such study cannot be freed from the warp of personal experience, the bias of individual prejudice, and above all, from the implication of prurience. And yet a certain measure of opprobrium would not be too great a price to pay in order to rid ourselves of many phallic fallacies.

From Dickinson in *JAMA*, 1925 and quoted in the preface of *Human Sexual Response* by Masters and Johnson in 1966.

Successful reproduction is the ultimate definition of evolutionary fitness. In humans, as in all mammals, fertilization occurs within the reproductive tract so intimate contact between male and female is necessary for spontaneous conception to occur. Mammalian sexual behavior is thus ultimately directed toward the physiology of coitus, which results in the deposition of sperm within the female reproductive tract.

For humans, however, a purely procreational approach to sexual behavior is too simplistic. Unlike most animals whose mating is seasonable and determined by hormonal cycles, humans and other primates are sexually receptive when they are not fertile. Human sexuality is thus defined not only by procreation but by recreation and pleasure. The non-reproductive aspect is quite plastic and subject to individual and cultural influences. What is pleasurable to one individual may not be so to another. Normative behavior in one culture may be unacceptable in another. What does seem to be common to all human sexual responses is that both physiologic and psychological satisfaction is central and motivating.

Most sexual encounters pass through a series of five stages, four of which were first defined by the pioneering work of Masters and Johnson. The first stage, sexual attraction or arousal, has been addressed more completely through the work of social psychologists interested in human sexuality. Although the validity of some of the data gathered by Masters and Johnson has been subject to question, their

model remains the single best description of the physiologic aspects of the human sexual response. Using hundreds of observations during heterosexual interactions and masturbation, they divided the human sexual response into excitement, plateau, orgasm and resolution phases.

Phases of the sexual response

Sexual attraction or arousal is the most individualized stage of the human sexual response. In many respects sexual attraction and arousal are closely tied to personality. They are also the most culturally determined. For example, incest taboos forbidding marriage and intercourse between closely related family members are almost universal among cultures over time, whereas attention to women's breasts or weight varies tremendously. Interestingly, two variables of attractiveness do appear both universal and related to reproductive success: youth and health.

Erotic stimuli can be quite varied and include mental images, smells, sounds and physical events such as touching or stroking. Men and women are about equally arousable as measured by both pelvic blood flow and by self-report, but differ dramatically in their preferences. Explicit visual stimuli such as body images and novel or unpredictable situations appeal to men more than women. Women generally prefer images with an emotional, romantic or familiar context. An individual's physical health and mental state contribute greatly to the threshold at which they can be aroused by a given stimulus.

During the physiologic **excitement phase**, sexual interest is stimulated by these psychological or physiologic stimuli. This aroused state then intensifies during the **plateau phase**. If stimulation is sufficient, **orgasm** or climax then occurs, typically as an explosive and pleasant release of sexual tension. Finally, during the **resolution phase**, sexual arousal dissipates and arousal and climacteric physiology reverts to baseline. Although both male and female progress through the same phases, they may differ in length and intensity in any one sexual encounter. The most notable physiologic difference between males and females is the presence of a refractory period in men during which sexual arousal cannot be restored and orgasm cannot occur. Women can be induced to orgasm from any point in the resolution phase with sufficient stimulation.

The basic physiologic responses of the human body to sexual stimulation are twofold. The primary reaction is **vascular congestion**. The secondary response is **generalized muscle tension** or myotonia. Reflexes activated within the spinal cord and modulated by higher central nervous system input control each response.

Male sexual response

The human male's first physiologic response to effective sexual stimulation is penile erection. During this excitement phase, vasodilatation of the lacunar smooth muscle of the penis leads to its engorgement and hardening (Chapter 12). Only a minimal degree of sexual tension may accompany excitation and this phase varies significantly in length.

Erectile stimuli may be either psychogenic or somatogenic. Psychogenic stimuli can include both imagined and direct visual cues such as explicitly erotic images. These signals are integrated within the limbic system of the brain and then transmitted via descending projections to the spinal cord where they travel via autonomic and visceral efferents to the penis. Somatogenic stimuli include touching the penis or adjacent perineum. These tactile stimuli will reflexly activate the same efferents as the spinal cord pathway does. This tactile reflex is typically preserved following spinal cord transection. The erection of the excitement phase may be quite susceptible to external signals and may be resolved without progression. Sudden loud noises including vocalizations and changes in the physical surroundings can impair penile erection in the excitation phase. Erection of the penis can also be elicited independently of the excitation phase of sexual arousal and has been observed in the newborn period and during sleep, especially in pubescent boys.

During the plateau phase, penile erection increases slightly as a minor involuntary increase in vasocongestion occurs. The scrotum and testes are drawn reflexly toward the perineum and the size of the testes increases secondarily to vasocongestion. Increases in both heart rate and systolic blood pressure occur. Immediately before ejaculation, a warm red rash may develop over the upper abdomen, trunk, neck and face. Diffuse muscular tension throughout the body is maximal. Muscular contractions within the prostate gland, vas deferens and seminal vesicles are induced and seminal plasma and spermatozoa are expelled into the posterior urethra. This process of **emission** is mediated by sympathetic output travelling through the hypogastric plexus and can be abolished by α-adrenergic blockade. Once the plateau phase is reached, detumescence without ejaculation and orgasm is rare in healthy individuals.

During orgasm, the somatic changes in the cardiovascular system are at their maximum, as is generalized muscle tension. Hyperventilation and vocalizations are common. Contraction of the smooth muscles of the urethra and the striated muscles of the bulbocavernosis and ischiocavernosus muscles expels the semen from the prostatic urethra. Both the pelvic floor and rectal sphincter may contract rhythmically. **Ejaculation** of the semen from the penis marks the height of orgasm. It is typically accompanied by release of sexual tension and an intense sense of pleasure.

Resolution phase penile detumescence occurs in two distinct stages. The primary stage of penile involution occurs very rapidly. The penis reduces in size from full erection to about 50% larger than its flaccid, unstimulated size. The penis is totally refractory to stimulation in this stage. Secondary stage involution is a more extended process

that returns the penis to its normal unstimulated size. The penis is only relatively refractory during this stage and progressively becomes excitable again with sufficient stimulation. Prolongation of the primary stage of detumescence occurs when the excitement or plateau phase of the sexual cycle is extended by voluntary efforts on the part of the male to delay ejaculation until his sexual partner is satisfied.

Female sexual response

During the excitement phase, somatogenic and psychogenic stimuli arouse the female through similar neural pathways to the male. The clitoral response to arousal is less predictable, however, than is that of its homolog, the penis. Tactile stimulation of the female perineum or the glans clitoris can elicit vasocongestion, engorgement of the body of the clitoris and erection only in some women. The excitement phase response of the vagina is much more predictable and consistent. Vaginal lubrication begins 10–30 s after receipt of arousing stimuli and continues progressively through orgasm. The longer the excitement and plateau phases, the greater the production of vaginal lubrication. During the excitement phase, the upper two-thirds of the vagina expands and lengthens, thereby elevating the uterus into the false pelvis. This repositioning elevates the cervix above the vaginal floor and 'tents' the midvaginal plane. These changes result in an increase in the circumference of the vaginal diameter, largely at the level of the cervix. Finally, during excitement the labia minora become markedly engorged with blood such that they displace the labia majora upward and outward away from the vaginal introitus. The increase in minor labial diameter adds at least 1 cm to the functional length of the vagina.

During the plateau phase, the most striking change in the female genitalia is florid coloration of the labia minora from congestion. This beet red appearance is the single most consistent physical marker for sexual arousal in the female. The clitoris retracts behind the hood formed by the labia. Hyperventilation and increased heart rate and blood pressure also develop late in the plateau phase; the magnitude of the change is not as marked in women as in men. Generalized myotonia may be present to the degree that carpopedal spasm, a spastic contraction of the striated muscle of the hands and feet, develops.

During coitus, penetration of the penis or other objects into the vagina can heighten a woman's sexual arousal by indirectly stimulating the retracted clitoris. This occurs because of traction on the engorged labia minora whose fused anterior segment forms the clitoral hood. Direct prolonged contact with the clitoris may actually be irritating, as the glans is extremely sensitive in the aroused state.

Orgasm in the female, like the male, involves rhythmic contractions of the reproductive organs followed by physical release from the vasocongestive and myotonic tension developed during arousal. Typically the contractions begin with the lower third of the vagina and evolve to encompass the entire vagina and uterus. A sex flush, which can also include diffuse fine perspiration, may develop over the woman's entire body.

Aside from ejaculation, there are two major physiologic differences between male and female orgasms. First, the female is capable of rapid return to another orgasm immediately following an orgasm, provided sexual stimulation occurs before she drops below plateau phase levels of arousal. Second, the female orgasm may last for a relatively long time compared to the male.

Finally, resolution involves decongestion of the labia, detumescence of the clitoris if it has occurred, and relaxation of the vagina.

15 Reproductive genetics

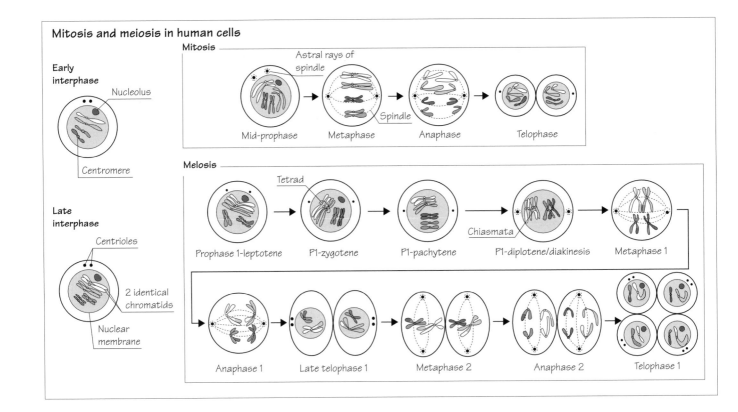

Mitosis and meiosis in human cells

Early interphase
- Nucleolus
- Centromere

Late interphase
- Centrioles
- 2 identical chromatids
- Nuclear membrane

Mitosis
- Astral rays of spindle
- Mid-prophase
- Metaphase
- Spindle
- Anaphase
- Telophase

Meiosis
- Tetrad
- Prophase 1-leptotene
- P1-zygotene
- P1-pachytene
- Chiasmata
- P1-diplotene/diakinesis
- Metaphase 1
- Anaphase 1
- Late telophase 1
- Metaphase 2
- Anaphase 2
- Telophase 1

Human chromosomes are complex structures consisting of deoxyribonucleic acid (DNA), ribonucleic acid (RNA) and protein. Each single helix of DNA is bounded at each end with a telomere, and has a centromere somewhere along the length of the chromosome. The function of the telomere is to protect the ends of the chromosome during DNA replication. The centromere is the site at which the mitotic spindle will attach and is necessary for proper segregation of the chromosomes during cell division. The centromere divides the chromosome into two arms that are identified as the p (petit) for the short arm and q for the long arm. The position of the centromere can be in the middle or anywhere along the arms. The positions of the centromeres have been used to group like chromosomes together as metacentric (central), distal (acrocentric) or others (submetacentric). The length of the chromosome plus the position of its centromere are used to identify individual chromosomes within the 22 pairs of autosomes and one pair of sex chromosomes (Chapter 5.1). The chromosomes are numbered in descending order of size, with number 1 the largest. The single exception to this rule are chromosomes 21 and 22 which are reversed so that 22 is larger than 21. Because of the historical convention of associating Down syndrome with trisomy 21, this pair of chromosomes was not renamed when the size difference became apparent. A karyotype is a display of chromosomes ordered from 1 to 22 plus the sex chromosomes, oriented so that the p arm is on the top. Females have a 46,XX karyotype and males a 46,XY karyotype.

Mitosis and meiosis, the two types of cell divisions, have several features in common. The first is the need to duplicate the entire chromosome content of the cell prior to division. Both use the cell machinery of the parent cell to make the DNA, RNA and new proteins that will participate in the cell division. Finally, both processes rely on use of the mitotic spindle to separate the chromosomes into the two poles of the cell destined to become the progeny of that cell. The major difference between mitosis and meiosis is that the duplicated chromosomes behave differently after DNA replication, thereby permitting the chromosome number of the daughter cells to be reduced from 46 to 23 by the end of meiosis. This reduction in chromosome number is necessary to convert the diploid (2N) germ cell precursors originating in the embryo into haploid (1N) germ cells, which will produce a new diploid organism at the time of fertilization.

During the **interphase** preceding cell division, the DNA for each chromosome is duplicated to 4N. As a result, each chromosome consists of two identical **chromatids** joined at the centromere. In mitosis, the chromosomes first shorten and thicken and the nucleoli and nuclear membrane break down (**prophase**). A mitotic spindle then forms between the two centrioles of the cell and all the chromosomes line up on its equator in **metaphase**. The centromere for each chromosome splits and one chromatid from each chromosome migrates to the polar ends of the mitotic spindle (**anaphase**). Finally, in **telophase**, new nucleoli and nuclear membranes form, the parent cell divides into two daughter cells and the mitotic spindle is disassembled. Two genetically identical cells now exist in place of the parent cell. **Mitosis is considered a non-sexual or vegetative form of reproduction.**

Meiosis involves two sequential cell divisions again beginning with the 4N DNA produced in interphase. In prophase of the first division (**prophase 1**), several specific and recognizable events occur. In the **leptotene** stage, the chromosomes become barely visible as the long thin structures they are in late interphase. Homologous pairs of chromosomes then come to lie side by side along parts of their length, forming tetrads (**zygotene** stage). The chromosomes thicken and shorten much as they do in mitotic prophase (**pachytene** stage); however, the pairing that took place in the zygotene stage permits **synapsis, crossing-over** and **chromatid exchange** to take place. In the **diplotene/diakinesis** stage, the chromosomes shorten even further. The paired homologous chromosomes show evidence of the crossing-over and chromatid exchange because of the chiasmata that join the arms of the chromosomes. Loops and unusual shapes within the chromosomes may be apparent at this stage. In **metaphase 1** of meiosis, the nuclear membrane breaks down and the joined pairs of homologous chromosomes line up at the equator of the spindle apparatus. One of each pair of homologous chromosomes then moves to each end of the cell along the spindle (**anaphase 1**). Nuclear membranes may then form, yielding two haploid daughter cells with 23 2N chromosomes in **telophase 1**. In the second meiotic division, these haploid cells then divide as if in mitosis. This second division produces four haploid cells each containing 23 1N chromosomes. **Unlike the cells produced in mitosis, these haploid germ cells are genetically unique and different from the parent cells because of the genetic exchanges that took place in the diplotene stage.** Haploid germ cells will participate in sexual reproduction in which a sperm cell and oocyte will come together to form a new diploid zygote.

While the sequence of events in meiosis during spermatogenesis and oogenesis is basically the same, there are also several important differences. In the prepubertal male, primordial germ cells are arrested in interphase. At puberty, these cells are reactivated to enter rounds of mitoses in the basal compartment of the seminiferous tubule. These reactivated cells are known as spermatogonial stem cells. From this reservoir of stem cells, type A spermatogonia emerge and divide several times again to produce a 'clone' of spermatogonia with identical genotypes. All of the spermatogonia from the clone then enter meiosis 1 and 2 to produce unique haploid sperm. New stem cells are constantly entering the spermatogenic cycle (Chapter 7) and thus the sperm supply is constantly renewing itself. Because of the relatively short time for spermatocytes to progress through meiosis and because of the tremendous competition among spermatozoa to reach the single oocyte within the female tract, fertilization of an egg by an aneuploid sperm is far rarer than the reverse.

In contrast to the testes, the ovary of a female at birth contains all the germ cells that it will ever have. These oocytes remain arrested in prophase 1 of meiosis until the LH surge at ovulation initiates metaphase 1. Thus, the duplicated genetic material in the oocyte sits paired with its homologous chromosome for anywhere from 10 to 50 years before the cell is called upon to divide. Oocytes are much more prone to chromosome abnormalities than are sperm for this reason. Failure of a pair of chromosomes to separate during meiosis is called **non-disjunction**. Non-disjunction can occur at either meiosis 1 or 2. When a single chromosome is involved, the aneuploid zygote is either **monosomic** or **trisomic** for the chromosome pair that failed to divide properly. Monosomic embryos, with the exception of monosomy X or Turner syndrome, are uniformly miscarried (Chapter 34.1). Most trisomic fetuses are also miscarried; only three (trisomy 13, 18 and 21) are reported among live births. If all the chromosomes are present in multiples of N, the embryo or fetus is **polyploid**.

Although it is critical that the zygote has 2N chromosomes, it is also important that one set of chromosomes comes from each parent. Cytogenetic studies of dermoid cysts and hydatidiform moles (gestational trophoblastic disease; Chapter 34.6) both of which have all 46 chromosomes from a single parent have demonstrated the importance of imprinting in early embryonic development. Imprinting is the process by which specific genes are methylated so that they can no longer be transcribed. Normal embryonic development requires that one set of genes be maternally imprinted and a second paternally. Otherwise, important steps in development will not occur and the zygote cannot form normally. If two sets of maternally imprinted genes are present, as happens in dermoid tumors of the ovary, disorganized fetal tissues without any supporting placenta or fetal membranes will develop. If two sets of paternally imprinted genes are present, as is found in hydatidiform moles, only dysplastic trophoblast and no fetus will develop. It is believed that maternal and paternal imprinting arose during the course of evolution to prevent self-fertilization in higher animal classes and thereby assure continued diversity in the gene pool.

16 Fertilization and the establishment of pregnancy

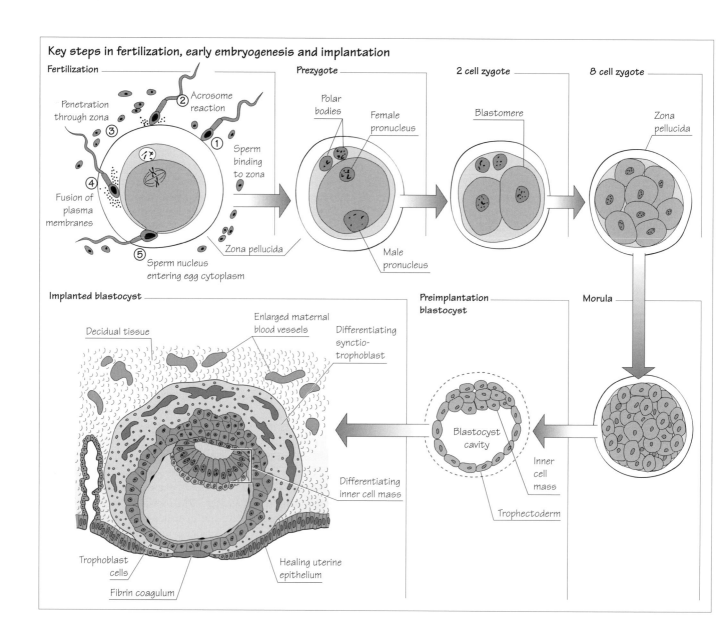

Key steps in fertilization, early embryogenesis and implantation

Fertilization

Penetration through zona

② Acrosome reaction

③

① Sperm binding to zona

④ Fusion of plasma membranes

⑤ Sperm nucleus entering egg cytoplasm

Zona pellucida

Prezygote

Polar bodies

Female pronucleus

Male pronucleus

2 cell zygote

Blastomere

8 cell zygote

Zona pellucida

Implanted blastocyst

Decidual tissue

Enlarged maternal blood vessels

Differentiating synctio-trophoblast

Trophoblast cells

Fibrin coagulum

Healing uterine epithelium

Differentiating inner cell mass

Preimplantation blastocyst

Blastocyst cavity

Inner cell mass

Trophectoderm

Morula

The egg

At ovulation, the egg is arrested in metaphase of the second meiotic division. It is surrounded by a proteinaceous ring called the **zona pellucida**. Granulosa cells that adhered to the surface of the zona and were expelled with the egg from the ovary remain attached as the cumulus. The sperm that ultimately fertilizes the egg must first negotiate these surrounding layers before it can penetrate the egg cell membrane at fertilization. The oocyte will remain viable for 6–24 h once ovulated.

The sperm

Within minutes of coitus, spermatozoa can be found in the cervix. The majority of sperm never enter the cervix but remain in the vagina where they eventually leak out as the semen first coagulates and then liquefies.

Those sperm that make it to the cervix can survive within the epithelial crypts for hours but cannot enter the uterus unless the cervical mucous is receptive. This typically occurs in midcycle when estrogen levels are high and progesterone low. The estrogen makes the cervix itself soft and its secretions thin and watery. Progesterone firms the cervix and makes its secretions tenacious and thick, hostile to spermatozoa.

Sperm movement through the uterus to the site of fertilization in the oviduct takes 2–7 h. It appears to result from a combination of ciliary beating by the uterine lining and the propulsive efforts of the sperm themselves. Abnormal sperm rarely can make this long trip successfully and even most of the healthy spermatozoa die along the way. Of the millions of sperm in a normal ejaculate, only several hundred will typically reach the oviducts. There they will linger in a quiet state until ovulation occurs. The spermatozoa then are reactivated and begin moving toward the egg. The signal that attracts the sperm to the egg is unknown. Human spermatozoa can survive 24–48 h total in the female reproductive tract.

Freshly ejaculated spermatozoa are not capable of fertilizing an egg. They must undergo a process known as **capacitation** before they are capable of penetrating the cell layers surrounding the oocyte. Capacitation typically occurs within the female reproductive tract, although the process can be induced *in vitro* under the proper culture conditions. Capacitation involves first removing a glycoprotein coat that adheres to the spermatozoa cell membranes. This initiates changes in the surface charge of the sperm membrane and reorganization of that membrane. Capacitated sperm change their tail movements from regular undulating waves to whip-like, thrashing movements that propel the sperm forward. At the biochemical level, capacitated sperm acquire increased calcium sensitivity and elevated internal cAMP levels. These latter biochemical changes are necessary before the sperm can undergo an acrosome reaction, which is the next step in the fertilization process. Capacitation takes several hours both *in vivo* and *in vitro*.

The **acrosome reaction** is crucial to the fertilization process because without it, the sperm is incapable of penetrating the zona pellucida. It begins when an intact, capacitated sperm comes in contact with the zona pellucida of an egg and binds through a specific glycoprotein, ZP3. ZP3 induces further calcium influx into the spermatozoa and cAMP increases further. The acrosome swells and its outer membrane fuses with the plasma membrane of the sperm. The contents of the acrosome are then released in the vicinity of the head of the sperm. Uncovering the inner acrosomal membrane exposes another zona binding protein, ZP2, that will hold the sperm close to the egg. Proteolytic enzymes released from the acrosome then facilitate penetration of the zona pellucida by the whiplashing sperm. Penetration of the zona takes about 15 min.

Fertilization

After the spermatozoa reaches the egg cell membrane, it fuses with it and almost immediately stops moving. The sperm nucleus enters the egg cytoplasm where it will form the male pronucleus.

Once the sperm and egg cell membranes fuse, three important events are triggered by a rise in intracellular calcium in the oocyte. The first is depolarization of the egg cell membrane, which prevents any other spermatozoa from fusing with it. This is the **primary block to polyspermy**. It assures that only one male pronucleus is available for fusion with the female pronucleus and protects the diploid status of the zygote. The second event is the fusion of a set of granules that lie just beneath the egg cell membrane with the membrane and their discharge into the zona pellucida. This reaction, known as the **cortical reaction**, serves to impair the ability of the zona to bind any more sperm. This is a **secondary block to polyspermy**. The third event is also involved in preserving a diploid zygote. This event is resumption of the second meiotic division of the egg. The second polar body is formed and extruded from the egg, thereby assuring that the female pronucleus is also haploid. Failure to preserve the diploid state of the conceptus is a frequent cause of early pregnancy failure (Chapter 34.1).

After the sperm has entered the egg, its cytoplasm mixes with that of the egg and the sperm nuclear membrane breaks down. A new membrane forms around the chromatin, forming the **male pronucleus**. Similarly, a new oocyte nuclear membrane forms around the **female pronucleus**. During this period, DNA synthesis begins as the haploid pronuclei prepare for the first mitotic division of the zygote. The pronu-

clear membranes break down, the parental chromosomes mix and then the metaphase mitotic spindle forms. The chromosomes separate and the first cell division occurs at about 24 h after fertilization.

Interestingly, although the spermatozoon induces remarkable changes in the oocyte at the time of fertilization, it is not necessary to activate the egg. Indeed, any event that stimulates an intracellular calcium rise will induce a cortical reaction and resumption of the second meiotic cell division. If the second polar body is either not formed or not expelled, a diploid activated egg develops. This abnormal self-activation is known as **parthenogenesis** and is the basis for the formation of dermoid cysts within the ovary (Chapter 39).

During the first few cell divisions, there is no new mRNA synthesis occurring from the nuclear DNA in the conceptus. The embryo stays the same total size with the size of each individual cell progressively becoming smaller. Thus, the embryo is developing using essentially only maternal cell components which has led to the observation that there are important signals passed on to the embryo through the oocyte cytoplasm. These signals likely reside in **mitochondrial DNA** which *is* replicated during early embryonic cell division. Mitochondrial DNA is stable and can be traced through generations to determine maternal lineage.

The establishment of pregnancy

Once fertilization has occurred, success of the pregnancy depends on implantation within the wall of the uterus and on signaling to the mother that pregnancy adaptations must occur. Without these two important events, the zygote will simply wash out of the uterus with the next menses.

The cleaving zygote will spend about one week floating in the oviduct as it progresses from the 16-cell stage through the solid **morula** (mulberry) stage and then becomes a 32–64-cell **blastocyst** by cavitating. At the time of blastocyst formation, the embryonic cells differentiate into two distinct types: the outer **trophectoderm** cells and the **inner cell mass**. The trophectoderm cells will eventually form the placenta while the inner cell mass will form the fetus and fetal membranes. It is at the blastocyst stage that the conceptus enters the uterus.

During the time that it spends in the oviduct, the conceptus remains surrounded by the zona pellucida. After about 2 days in the uterus, the blastocyst will first attach to, and then invade, the endometrial lining of the uterus. In order to have its cells make contact with the endometrium, the blastocyst must lose or 'hatch' from the zona pellucida. Simultaneously, the trophectodermal cells of the blastocyst begin to differentiate into **trophoblast** cells which make contact with the luminal epithelial cells. Within hours, the surface epithelium immediately underlying the conceptus becomes eroded and nearby cells lyse, releasing primary metabolic substrates for use by the blastocyst. The endometrium undergoes dramatic biochemical and morphologic changes called **decidualization**. Decidualization begins at the point of attachment and spreads out in a concentric wave from the point of implantation. The endometrium begins to heal over the conceptus so that the entire implantation becomes buried within the endometrium or **interstitial** in location.

Invasion then involves further differentiation of the trophoblast cells into two cell types: the **cytotrophoblasts** and the **syncytiotrophoblasts**. Syncytiotrophoblasts are large, multinucleated cells that develop from cytotrophoblasts and acquire invasive properties. The syncytiotrophoblasts invade both the endometrial stroma and blood vessels they unroof to form vascular lacunae. Eventually the syncytiotrophoblasts will reach and invade the spiral arteries of the endometrium. Appropriate invasion of the spiral arteries is key to a normal pregnancy outcome (Chapter 34.5).

A number of growth factors involved in implantation have been identified. These include: (i) leukaemia inhibitory factor, a cytokine; (ii) the integrins, which mediate cell–cell interactions; (iii) transforming growth factor beta (TGF-β), which stimulates synctium formation and inhibits trophoblast invasion; and (iv) epidermal growth factor and (v) interleukin 1β, both of which mediate trophoblast invasion.

Implantation occurs about 7–10 days after ovulation. If the conceptus is to survive beyond day 14 post ovulation in the uterus, the corpus luteum must continue to secrete progesterone. **Human chorionic gonadotropin** (hCG) produced by the developing trophoblast and secreted into the maternal bloodstream acts like luteinizing hormone on the corpus luteum and ensures that luteal regression will not occur (Chapter 17).

Endocrinology of pregnancy

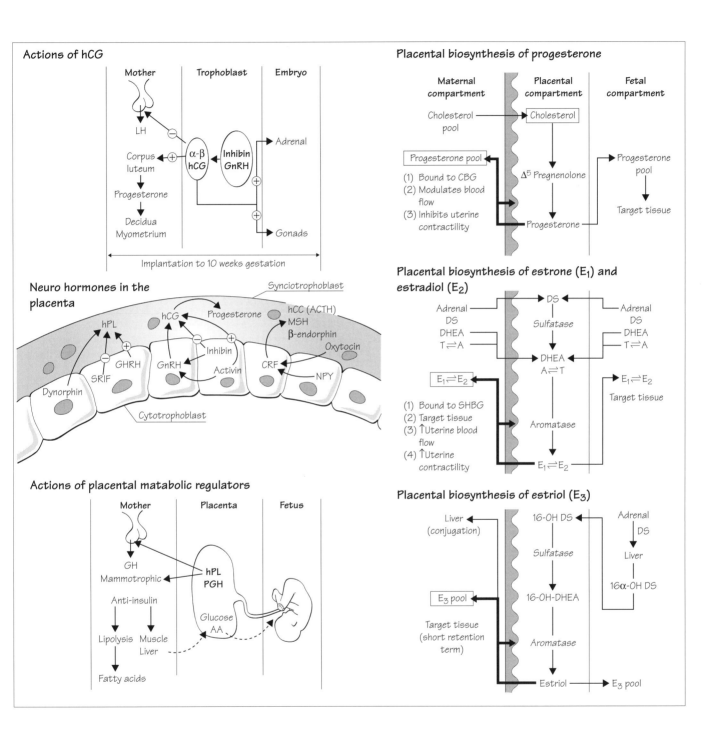

Actions of hCG

Mother | Trophoblast | Embryo

Implantation to 10 weeks gestation

Neuro hormones in the placenta

Synciotrophoblast

Cytotrophoblast

Actions of placental matabolic regulators

Mother | Placenta | Fetus

Placental biosynthesis of progesterone

Maternal compartment | Placental compartment | Fetal compartment

(1) Bound to CBG
(2) Modulates blood flow
(3) Inhibits uterine contractility

Placental biosynthesis of estrone (E_1) and estradiol (E_2)

(1) Bound to SHBG
(2) Target tissue
(3) ↑Uterine blood flow
(4) ↑Uterine contractility

Placental biosynthesis of estriol (E_3)

The placenta is a very rich source of both steroid and protein hormones, only a few of which are unique to pregnancy. These placental hormones are responsible for almost all the maternal and some of the fetal adaptations to pregnancy.

Human chorionic gonadotropin

Human chorionic gonadotropin (hCG) is a dimeric protein hormone whose structure is closely related to luteinizing hormone (LH) (Chapter 2). It is among the earliest products of the trophoblast cells of the embryo and is a necessary signal to the maternal organism indicating conception. β-hCG mRNA can be detected as early as the 8-cell stage but intact hCG is not detectable in the maternal bloodstream or urine until 6 days after fertilization. hCG secretion is quantitatively related to the total mass of cytotrophoblast in the placenta. Its concentration in the maternal serum doubles every 2–3 days in early pregnancy; this can be used as a screen to differentiate normal from abnormal pregnancies. Failure of the hCG concentrations to double as expected may indicate an abnormal implantation such as an ectopic (tubal) pregnancy or a non-viable intrauterine gestation. Higher than expected levels of hCG are seen with multiple gestations and molar pregnancies.

The major biologic role of hCG is to 'rescue' the corpus luteum of the ovary from its programmed demise 12–14 days after ovulation. Because of the close structural relationship of hCG to LH, hCG is able to bind to the LH receptor on the luteal cells. This results in maintenance of the corpus luteum, continued secretion of ovarian progesterone after day 14 and maintenance of the early pregnancy. Surgical removal of the corpus luteum without progesterone supplementation or administration of an antiprogestin such as RU-486 before the 9th menstrual week of pregnancy will result in a pregnancy loss. Subsequent to week 9, progesterone production is taken over by the placenta which now has sufficient mass to support production of the large amount of progesterone necessary for pregnancy maintenance. At the end of the first trimester, hCG also stimulates the fetal gonads to make steroid hormones that are responsible for differentiation of the internal and external genitalia (Chapter 5).

hCG secretion, like that of many of the hormones produced within the placenta, appears to occur in a two-cell model that mimics the interactions between the neuroendocrine hypothalamus and the pituitary. Thus, gonadotropin-releasing hormone (GnRH) secreted by the cytotrophoblast stimulates hCG production by the syncytiotrophoblast. As pregnancy progresses and the placenta becomes the major site of progesterone production, hCG's primary role changes from maintenance of the corpus luteum to maintenance of progesterone production by the syncytiotrophoblast. The serum level of hCG reflects this change by increasing to a maximum at about the 7th menstrual week of pregnancy and then decreasing to a much lower steady state level for the remainder of the pregnancy.

Progesterone and estrogens

Progesterone production by the syncytiotrophoblast is dependent on maternal substrate in the form of circulating low-density lipoprotein cholesterol. Unlike other steroid producing glands, the placenta lacks the enzymes to form cholesterol from acetate as can be done in the other steroid-forming glands. hCG regulates the synthesis and secretion of progesterone. Very large amounts of progesterone are produced and secreted into the maternal bloodstream. The progesterone is active locally within the uterus where it acts both to maintain the decidual lining of the uterus and as a potent relaxant upon the smooth muscle cells of the myometrium. It also has peripheral effects upon vascular smooth muscle and other organs that must adapt to the demands of pregnancy (Chapter 18).

The placenta also expresses abundant amounts of the enzyme aromatase, which is responsible for converting androgens to **estrogens**. All three estrogens, estradiol (E_2), estrone (E_1) and estriol (E_3) are produced in the placenta although the sources of the androgen precursors are different for the three. The aromatase is not rate-limiting, so that the amount of estrogen produced is determined by the amount of substrate delivered to the placenta. The major androgen precursor in placental estrogen production is dehydroepiandrosterone sulfate (DHEA-S) which is an adrenal androgen. The placenta has an abundance of the sulfate-cleaving enzyme sulfatase, which converts DHEA-S to DHEA. Maternal DHEA-S is all converted to DHEA, then to androstenedione, then testosterone and finally to estrone and estradiol (Chapter 3). Some

fetal DHEA-S is converted to estrone and estradiol, but the majority of it is converted to estriol, an estrogen not made by the ovary. Most of the fetal DHEA-S undergoes 16-hydroxylation in the fetal liver. When the fetal 16-OH-DHEA-S reaches the placenta, the placental sulfatase cleaves the sulfate side chain and then it is further metabolized and aromatized to estriol. The amount of estriol produced by the placenta far exceeds that of estrone and estradiol, making placental **estriol** of fetal origin the major placental estrogen.

Like progesterone, most of the estrogen produced by the placenta is found in the maternal compartment (uterus and bloodstream). While estriol is a weak estrogen by comparison to estradiol and estrone, it appears to be as effective as these two more potent estrogens in increasing uteroplacental blood flow. Thus its relatively weak estrogenic effects on other organ systems make it highly effective in this single important pregnancy function. Its unique production from a fetal substrate also permits fetal regulation of uteroplacental blood flow, an important determinant of fetal growth and well-being.

Human placental lactogen

Human placental lactogen (hPL) is a protein hormone produced exclusively by the placenta that is closely related to both prolactin and growth hormone (GH). When the peptide was originally isolated from the placenta, its biologic activity was assessed in animal models where it has lactogenic activity and hence it was designated as a lactogen. Whether it has lactogenic activity in the human remains unknown. Instead it appears to be a metabolic hormone with activities closely related to those of GH with which it shares 96% structural homology. Another name for hPL is **human chorionic somatomammotropin (hCS)**.

hCS production is directly proportional to placental mass and, therefore, rises steadily throughout pregnancy. Prolonged fasting and hypoglycemia increase its production. The amount of this hormone produced at term (>1 g/day) is the largest amount of any protein hormone in either men or women.

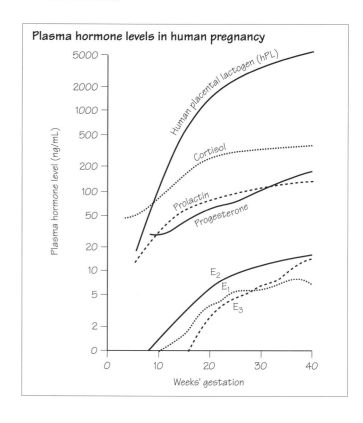

The exact function of hPL is not known because successful pregnancies have been reported in the absence of hPL production by the placenta. However, there is growing evidence that hPL is involved in regulating glucose homeostasis in the mother such that she can meet the nutritional demands of the fetus. The effects of hPL on fat and carbohydrate metabolism are similar to those seen with GH and include inhibition of peripheral glucose uptake, stimulation of insulin release by the pancreas and an increase in plasma free fatty acids. During pregnancy, blood glucose decreases and insulin secretion increases, as does peripheral insulin resistance consistent with GH-like activity. In theory, the decreased maternal glucose utilization induced by hPL would ensure that a steady supply of glucose is available for fetal utilization.

Other hormones

A placental variant of the pituitary growth hormone known as **PGH** has been identified. Pituitary growth hormone of either maternal or fetal origin is not necessary for normal fetal growth because anencephalic fetuses lacking a pituitary gland and the offspring of women with growth hormone deficiency grow normally *in utero*, PGH is a candidate hormone for regulating fetal growth.

Both the cytotrophoblast and syncytiotrophoblast secrete **corticotropin-releasing hormone (CRH)** and **pro-opiomelanocortin (POM-C)**, the precursor of **adrenocorticotropic hormone (ACTH)**. Maternal CRH levels and placental CRH content rise in the last month of pregnancy. Glucocorticoids enhance CRH mRNA production suggesting a positive feedback system. It is hypothesized that placental CRH and ACTH may be involved in the timing of the onset of parturition.

18 Maternal adaptations to pregnancy

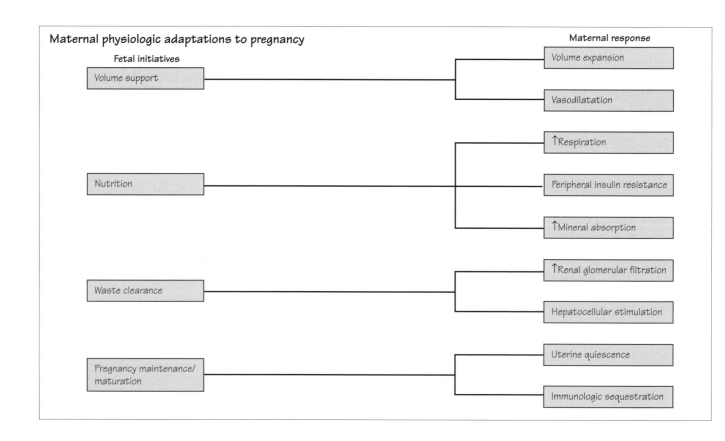

Maternal physiologic adaptations to pregnancy

Fetal initiatives	Maternal response
Volume support	Volume expansion
	Vasodilatation
Nutrition	↑Respiration
	Peripheral insulin resistance
	↑Mineral absorption
Waste clearance	↑Renal glomerular filtration
	Hepatocellular stimulation
Pregnancy maintenance/ maturation	Uterine quiescence
	Immunologic sequestration

Adaptations occur in the mother in response to a series of needs created by the pregnancy. These include fetal support in the form of increasing volume for the fetus and amniotic fluid, nutrition for the fetus and placenta in the form of glucose, amino acids and oxygen, clearance of fetal waste, and protection for the fetus from perturbations in the system such as starvation or drugs. In addition, there is a need for the timely onset of labor, for the protection of the mother from cardiovascular insults at the time of delivery and preparation for the extrauterine nourishment of the infant. All maternal systems are affected to some degree.

Cardiovascular system

During the first two trimesters there is an increase in the circulating blood volume of 40% (3500 cc expands to 5000 cc). This occurs via upregulation of the renin–angiotensin system. Placental estrogen increases the hepatic production of angiotensinogen and estrogen and progesterone together increase the production of the proteolytic enzyme, renin, by the kidney. Renin cleaves the angiotensinogen to form angiotensin I, which is then converted into angiotensin II (AII) in the lung and elsewhere. The increased AII acts on the zona glomerulosa of the adrenal to increase aldosterone production. Aldosterone favors volume expansion through sodium and water retention. Iron absorption increases to meet the demand for increased hemoglobin during the volume expansion.

Concomitant with the increase in circulating blood volume is a loss of peripheral vascular responsiveness to AII, a potent vasoconstrictor. This results in a drop in blood pressure during the early second trimester in most women in spite of the higher AII levels. Blood pressures gradually rise to prepregnancy levels by the third trimester. Progesterone also mediates some of the changes in blood pressure.

Respiratory system

An increase in tidal volume, minute ventilatory volume and minute O_2 uptake develops in pregnant women. These result in increased oxygen delivery to the periphery and in a mild respiratory alkalosis that is compensated for by increased renal bicarbonate excretion. There is some evidence that progesterone is responsible for these changes. The kinetics of O_2 association with fetal hemoglobin favor O_2 unloading to the fetus in the placenta.

Many pregnant women have the sensation of shortness of breath in the absence of pathology for reasons that still remain unclear.

Kidney and urinary tract

The glomerular filtration rate (GFR) and renal plasma flow (RPF) increase, beginning in early pregnancy. GFR increases as much as 50% by midpregnancy and remains elevated, whereas RPF begins to decrease in the third trimester. Therefore the filtration fraction increases in the last third of pregnancy. Because of the increased GFR, serum creatinine and urea are lower in pregnancy than in the non-pregnant state and creatinine clearance is increased.

An increase in the filtered load of sodium by 60–70% occurs with the increased GFR. Progesterone appears to cause some sodium wastage by interfering with normal sodium resorption in the proximal tubule. Aldosterone increases proportionately to 2–3 times normal.

Reabsorption of glucose in the proximal tubule is decreased because of a relatively fixed tubular reabsorptive capacity in the face of the increased GFR. Glucose is detectable in the urine of about 15% of normal pregnant women, but any woman exhibiting glycosuria should be evaluated for diabetes.

The volume of urine contained in the renal pelves and ureters can double in the latter half of pregnancy because of dilatation of the collecting system. This appears to result from both mechanical obstruction by the pregnant uterus and the relaxing effects of progesterone upon smooth muscle. This dilatation and resultant stagnation increases the risk of developing acute kidney infections during pregnancy.

Gastrointestinal tract and metabolism

A state of relative hyperinsulinism with peripheral insulin resistance develops during pregnancy. Pregnancy therefore is a potentially diabetogenic state. The high levels of estrogen, progesterone and placental lactogen (hPL) appear to cause hypertrophy, hyperplasia and hypersecretion of the beta islet cells of the pancreas; however, many pregnant women show prolonged hyperglycemia after meals in spite of the rise in insulin secretion. This observation, along with three others: (i) exaggerated insulin release in response to glucose infusion; (ii) reduced peripheral uptake of glucose; and (iii) suppressed glucagon secretion, has led to the conclusion that peripheral insulin resistance is present in pregnancy. The mechanism(s) for insulin resistance are not well understood. hPL with its growth hormone-like activity may be responsible. hPL may also promote lipolysis and liberation of free fatty acids which facilitates tissue resistance to insulin. The mechanisms above ensure a continuous supply of glucose for transfer to the fetus; however, they also produces an 'accelerated starvation' profile in the fasted pregnant woman. Fasted pregnant women are relatively hypoglycemic and have higher circulating free fatty acids, triglycerides and cholesterol. Prolonged fasting or persistent vomiting in pregnant women can rapidly lead to ketonemia.

Increased synthesis of hepatic proteins including procoagulants, bile acids and steroid precursors occurs and the cytochrome P450 oxidative pathway in the liver is stimulated. High circulating estrogens are responsible for these changes. The procoagulants most markedly elevated are Factors I (fibrinogen), VII, VIII, IX and X. The higher concentrations of clotting cascade proteins protect the mother from excessive blood loss at the time of delivery; however, they also predispose pregnant and postpartum women to an increased risk of venous thrombosis and embolism. The increased activity of the P450 system can dramatically alter drug metabolism, necessitating careful monitoring of plasma drug levels of commonly used therapeutics such as anticonvulsants and antibiotics in pregnant women.

Calcium absorption in the intestine increases. The calcium requirements of the developing fetal and neonatal skeleton produce a profound calcium stress during pregnancy and lactation. Plasma parathyroid hormone (PTH) concentrations rise despite a minimal decrease in circulating free calcium. Intestinal absorption of calcium is enhanced by increased circulating 1,25-dihydroxyvitamin D_3, the active metabolite of vitamin D. 1,25-$(OH)_2$-D_3 increases both because PTH increases

hepatic synthesis of 25-(OH)-D_3 and because the activity of the final converting enzyme 1α-hydroxylase increases in pregnancy. In non-pregnant women and men, conversion of 25-(OH)-D_3 to the 1,25 active form is limited by the activity of 1α-hydroxylase, which is found only in the kidney. In pregnant patients, 1α-hydroxylase is produced by both the decidua and placenta, thereby assuring an adequate amount of active D_3 to optimize dietary calcium absorption during pregnancy. If dietary calcium intake is adequate, minimal mobilization of maternal bone calcium occurs; otherwise fetal and neonatal skeletal mineralization will proceed at the expense of the maternal bone density.

Relaxation of all parts of the gastrointestinal (GI) tract occurs because of the effects of progesterone on smooth muscle. Gastric emptying is delayed as well as movement of digested material all along the tract. Gallbladder emptying is slower and bile tends to sludge in the bile duct and common duct.

Minor disorders of the GI tract including nausea, vomiting, constipation and heartburn are very common in pregnancy.

Hematologic system

The total red cell mass increases as the maternal intravascular volume increases, although to a lesser degree. This results in the development of a mild dilutional anemia. This dilutional anemia protects the mother from excess hemoglobin loss at delivery. The exact mechanism by which the anemia develops is not clear. Erythropoietin production is increased, but red cell mass does not increase in direct proportion to the increase in intravascular fluid volume. Accompanying this increase in total red cell mass is a requirement for sufficient iron to satisfy both maternal and fetal red cell production. The iron requirements of normal pregnancy are about 1.0 g, most of which is needed in the second half of pregnancy. The amount of iron absorbed from the diet alone, as well as any mobilized from maternal stores, may be insufficient to meet the demand.

A modest leucocytosis develops during pregnancy which can become quite marked during labor and postpartum. The reason for the early pregnancy change is unknown. During labor, the leucocytosis resembles that seen with strenuous exercise when previously sequestered white cells reenter the active circulation.

Increased coagulability develops because of the increased procoagulant synthesis in the liver. Up to 8% of women will develop a mild thrombocytopenia (<150 000 platelets/μL) which does not result in a bleeding diathesis. The mechanism by which the thrombocytopenia develops is unknown.

Endocrine system

Elevated circulating estrogen causes an increase in thyroid binding globulin (TBG) as part of the overall stimulation of hepatic proteins. This leaves less thyroid hormone free to circulate and hypothalamic TRH increases in response. TSH is then increased and the thyroid gland stimulated to produce sufficiently more T_3 and T_4 to return the circulating levels to normal. Pregnant women therefore have higher levels of TBG, total T_3 and T_4, but normal amounts of free T_3 and T_4. This can cause confusion when interpreting thyroid function tests in pregnancy. It also means that pregnant women taking hormone replacement for thyroid gland deficiency often need to increase their dose to maintain adequate free hormone levels.

Aldosterone and cortisol secretion are both increased during pregnancy. Pituitary production of prolactin increases dramatically as a result of estrogen stimulation. The number of lactotrophs in the pituitary doubles, thereby almost doubling the size and blood supply of the pituitary gland. This increase in size makes the pituitary gland particularly vulnerable to ischemic damage if postpartum hemorrhage and shock are not promptly treated (Sheehan syndrome).

Immune system

Cellular immunity decreases during pregnancy, probably as a compensatory mechanism to permit the mother to tolerate the fetal allograft. Unique trophoblast antigens have been recently identified, as has the absence of major histocompatibility class II antigens on the surface of trophoblast. A clinical correlate of the altered immune response is that pregnant women are more susceptible to viral infections, experiencing a higher attack rate and more severe or prolonged disease.

Skin

Circulating melanotrophic hormone (MSH) is increased as a result of the increased production of the precursor molecule POM-C (Chapter 17). MSH causes darkening on the skin across the cheeks (chloasma or pregnancy mask) and darkening of the linea alba, the slightly pigmented line on the skin that runs from the navel to the pubis. Hair may also appear to fall out in clumps because of synchronization of hair follicle growth cycles during pregnancy.

Labor

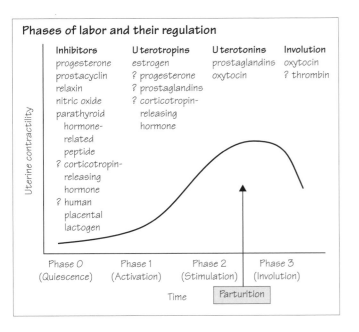

Phases of labor and their regulation

Inhibitors	Uterotropins	Uterotonins	Involution
progesterone	estrogen	prostaglandins	oxytocin
prostacyclin	? progesterone	oxytocin	? thrombin
relaxin	? prostaglandins		
nitric oxide	? corticotropin-		
parathyroid	releasing		
hormone-	hormone		
related			
peptide			
? corticotropin-			
releasing			
hormone			
? human			
placental			
lactogen			

Phase 0 (Quiescence)   Phase 1 (Activation)   Phase 2 (Stimulation)   Phase 3 (Involution)

Time   Parturition

Uterine contractility

Labor is the process by which the fetus and its supporting placenta and membranes pass from the uterus to the outside world. **It is defined as regular uterine contractions that result in thinning and dilatation of the cervix so that the products of conception can pass out of the uterus.** Labor involves three key processes: (i) a switch in myometrial activity from a longer-lasting, low-frequency contraction pattern called 'contractures' to the frequent, high-intensity and regular pattern known as 'contractions'; (ii) softening and dilatation of the cervix; and (iii) rupture of the fetal membranes. Although labor may become apparent with the appearance of any of these three elements, typically the physiologic events that produce them all occur simultaneously.

Phases of labor

For simplicity, the term labor is best thought of as occuring in four physiologic phases that represent the process of labor as a release of the myometrium from the inhibitory effects of pregnancy, along with the activation of stimulants of myometrial contractility. During Phase 0, or pregnancy, the uterus is in a state of quiescence which is induced by one or more inhibitors. Candidate inhibitors include progesterone, prostacyclin, nitric oxide, parathyroid hormone-related peptide (PTHrP), calcitonin gene-related peptide, relaxin, adrenomedullin and vasoactive intestinal peptide (VIP). Near term, the uterus undergoes the process of activation (Phase 1). During activation, a number of contraction-associated proteins increase under the influence of estrogen. These proteins include myometrial receptors for prostaglandins and oxytocin, membranous ion channels and connexin-43, a key component of gap junctions. These new gap junctions will electrically couple adjacent myometrial cells, thereby permitting maximum coordination of waves of contractions from the fundus to the cervix. Following Phase 1 activa-

tion, Phase 2 or stimulation occurs. During stimulation, oxytocin and stimulatory prostaglandins (PGs) such as PGE_2 and $PGF_{2\alpha}$ can induce contractions in the primed uterus. During Phase 2, the cervix dilates and at parturition, the fetus, membranes and placenta are expelled from the uterus. Phase 3 is the sustained contraction of the uterus that is necessary to provide hemostasis and eventually to reduce the enlarged postpartum uterus back to its non-pregnant state, a process called involution.

Initiation of labor

The average human gestation lasts 280 days (40 weeks) from the beginning of the last menstrual period. Exactly what triggers human labor is unknown. The best available evidence suggests that in all species that bear live young, the fetoplacental unit controls at what point in gestation labor will occur and the mother determines the time of day that it will start. The mechanisms that the fetoplacental unit uses to signal the mother to start labor vary from species to species. Early studies using non-primate species such as sheep, rats and mice led to false assumptions about the physiology of human labor. Now, most of what we assume happens in human labor is extrapolated from other primates.

In primates, the initiation of labor does not involve progesterone withdrawal to the extent that it does in sheep and rodents. Instead, initiation of labor in primates appears to involve an increase in estrogen synthesis in the placenta. The sources of the increased estrogen include both an increase in production of adrenal androgen precursor (androstenedione) from the fetus and a stimulation of placental aromatase activity (Chapter 17). It appears that estrogen production in the placenta is key because systemic infusion of estrogen does not induce labor at term in spite of data showing a longitudinal rise in estrogen concentrations immediately preceding labor in all primate species. Infused androstenedione will induce contractions that can be blocked with an inhibitor of aromatase activity.

The stimulus to the increased fetal adrenal androgen production near term is not known. Experiments of nature where the fetus lacks a pituitary gland (anencephaly) have shown that these pregnancies are not abnormally prolonged. The most likely source of the stimulus is corticotropin-releasing factor (CRH) produced by the placenta. Placental CRH is biochemically identical to hypothalamic CRH but differs in its regulation. In contrast to the negative feedback glucocorticoids have on hypothalamic CRH, placental CRH is stimulated by glucocorticoids. This CRH probably has multiple loci of action including the fetal pituitary gland where it stimulates ACTH production and fetal adrenal steroid synthesis leading to increased androstenedione production. Placental CRH appears also to have local effects within the uterus, which include placental vasodilatation, prostaglandin production and myometrial contractility.

Whatever the stimulus is that *initiates* labor in humans and other primates, the cascade of events within the myometrium that leads to contractions is better understood. The final common pathway in labor in all species appears to be an increase in prostaglandin synthesis, notably PGE and PGF, by the decidua and the fetal membranes. Human uterine tissues are selectively enriched with arachidonic acid, an essential fatty acid that is the obligate precursor of these PGs. The cyclo-oxygenase

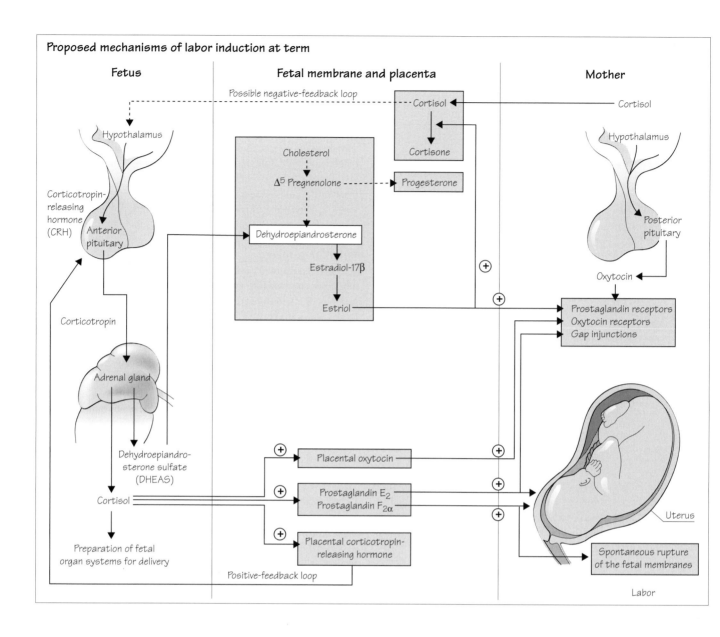

Proposed mechanisms of labor induction at term

enzymes, COX-1 and COX-2, are both expressed in the uterus; COX-2, the inducible form of the enzyme, appears to be sensitive to glucocorticoid induction. Evidence for the role of prostaglandins includes observations that: (i) the concentrations of PGs in amniotic fluid, maternal plasma and maternal urine are increased just prior to the onset of labor; (ii) administration of PGs at any stage of pregnancy has the capacity to initiate labor; (iii) PGs can induce cervical ripening, contractions and increase myometrial sensitivity to oxytocin; and (iv) inhibitors of PG synthesis, such as the COX inhibitor indometacin, can suppress contractions and prolong pregnancy.

Myometrial cells, like other smooth muscle cells, are triggered to contract by a rise in intracellular calcium (Ca^{2+}). Prostaglandins raise Ca^{2+} by increasing Ca^{2+} influx across the cell membranes, stimulating calcium release from intracellular stores and enhancing myometrial gap junction formation.

The posterior pituitary hormone, oxytocin, plays at least two roles in labor. Oxytocin acts through its receptor to activate members of the G-protein subfamily that acts through phospholipase C and inositol triphosphate to release intracellular Ca^{2+}. The increase in intracellular calcium mediates the effects of the oxytocin. The best known role of oxytocin is in assisting expulsion of the fetus during the second stage of labor after the cervix is fully dilated. However, oxytocin also appears to play a role in determining the time of day that labor will start, which is a maternally derived signal. Several days to weeks before the onset of recognizable labor, a switch occurs in myometrial activity away from contractures to contractions. This switch in myometrial activity invariably occurs when the lights go off in the animal's environment thereby ensuring that delivery will occur when the mother is safely at rest away from predators. Nocturnally active animals will thus deliver during the day and vice versa. This circadian rhythm of uterine activity is accompanied by an increase in both circulating oxytocin and myometrial oxytocin receptors.

A third role for oxytocin may be in the actual initiation of labor. While oxytocin can be used clinically to both induce and stimulate labor, the oxytocin concentrations in the maternal circulation do not begin to rise until the expulsive stage of labor begins. This finding originally led to doubt that the hormone was involved in the actual onset of labor. There is, however, a gradual increase in the concentrations of oxytocin receptor in the myometrium in the second half of pregnancy. Interestingly, the fetus, placenta and fetal membranes all make oxytocin that is selectively secreted toward the maternal compartment. Oxytocin can induce prostaglandin production and gap junction formation within the uterus, suggesting that it may act in synergy with other factors to begin labor.

20 The breast and lactation

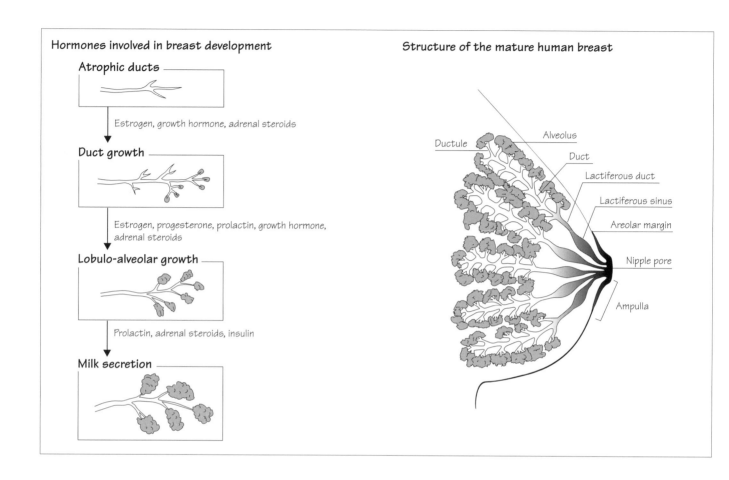

Hormones involved in breast development

Atrophic ducts

↓ Estrogen, growth hormone, adrenal steroids

Duct growth

↓ Estrogen, progesterone, prolactin, growth hormone, adrenal steroids

Lobulo-alveolar growth

↓ Prolactin, adrenal steroids, insulin

Milk secretion

Structure of the mature human breast

Ductule · Alveolus · Duct · Lactiferous duct · Lactiferous sinus · Areolar margin · Nipple pore · Ampulla

Development of the breast

The human mammary gland is derived from ectoderm. It is first visible in the 4-week embryo as a bud or nodule of epithelial tissue which appears along a line known as the milk crest. This line extends from the midaxilla to the inguinal region in the more developed embryo and may be the site of supernumary breasts or nipples in the adult. The epithelial nodule becomes buried in embryonic mesenchyme where the nodule undergoes further differentiation, apparently under the influence of paracrine signals from the mesenchyme. Secondary epithelial buds form cellular cords that elongate, bifurcate and hollow out. These cords become the excretory and lactiferous ducts of the mammary gland.

The human mammary gland is a compound tuboalveolar structure composed of 15–25 irregular lobes radiating out from the nipple. The lobes are separated by a dense layer of connective tissue and embedded in adipose tissue. Each lobe is further subdivided into a series of lobules that are connected to the nipple by lactiferous ducts. The lactiferous ducts are lined by a stratified squamous epithelium. Loose connective tissue (stroma) surrounds the ducts permitting the ducts to distend easily during lactation.

At birth, the breast is rudimentary and consists almost entirely of lactiferous ducts. Although the newborn breast may secrete a few drops of milk called 'witch's milk', this secretory function is short-lived and the breast becomes quiescent until puberty. At puberty, ovarian estrogens stimulate the lactiferous duct system to grow. After menarche, cyclic progesterone exposure induces further ductal growth as well as the development of rudimentary lobules at the ends of the ducts. Ductal epithelium remains sensitive to estrogen stimulation and the stroma, to progesterone stimulation through a woman's reproductive years. The breasts will continue to grow for several years after menarche as the lactiferous ducts progressively subdivide, elongate and hollow out and adipose tissue accumulates. However, lobular development will not proceed beyond a rudimentary stage in the absence of pregnancy.

At the beginning of pregnancy there is rapid growth and branching of the terminal portions of the rudimentary lobules. Vascularity increases dramatically. These two changes are often perceived shortly after conception by a woman as a 'tingling' or 'tension' in her breasts that will last for the first trimester. At about 8 menstrual weeks of pregnancy, true alveolar differentiation will begin. True glandular acini will appear as hollow alveoli lined with a single layer of myoepithelial cells. The highly branched myoepithelial cells will form a loose network surrounding the alveoli, which connect to the larger lactiferous ducts through intralobular ducts. Alveolar secretion begins during the second trimester and by the third trimester, an immunoglobulin-rich secretion is seen distending the alveoli.

While the role of ovarian steroids in breast development is clearly established on clinical grounds (prepubertal gonadal failure is associated with absence of breast development), other hormones have been implicated in human breast development based on animal models. Insulin is involved in multiplication of epithelial cells and formation of lobuloalveolar architecture. Complete cytologic and functional differentiation of the epithelial cells lining the alveoli requires cortisol, insulin and prolactin. Other growth factors such as insulin-like growth factor I (IGF-I) and epidermal growth factor (EGF) may be involved, as receptors for both of these have been demonstrated on mammary cells.

Milk formation

Milk is a complex food composed of more than 100 constituents. It is basically an emulsion of fat in a liquid phase that is isotonic with plasma. Mature human milk contains 3–5% fat, 1% protein, 7% lactose and 0.2% minerals and delivers 60–75 kcal/dL. The principal class of human milk lipids is triglyerides, of which palmitic and oleic acids are the most common. The principal proteins in milk are casein, α-lactalbumin, lactoferrin, immunoglobulin A, lysozyme and albumin. Casein and α-lactalbumin are specific milk proteins; α-lactalbumin is part of the enzyme complex lactose synthetase. Free amino acids, urea, creatinine and creatine are present. Lactose is the principal sugar. The protein content is higher in colostrum, the first milk, and the sugar content is lower. Minerals include sodium, potassium, calcium, magnesium, phosphorus and chloride. As the composition of human breast milk continues to be studied, a number of peptide hormones, including epidermal growth factor (EGF), transforming growth factor α (TGF-α), somatostatin and the insulin-like growth factors I and II (IGF-I and IGF-II) have been identified in the milk as well as the above nutrients.

The alveolar epithelial cells that make milk are polarized, highly differentiated cells whose function is to accumulate, synthesize, package and export the components of milk. **Milk formation includes at least four transcellular pathways** within the alveolus of the breast. The first pathway involves **secretion of monovalent cations and water**. Water moves across the cell drawn by a concentration gradient generated by the specific milk sugar, lactose, while the ions follow an electrochemical gradient. The second pathway is **receptor-mediated transport of immunoglobulins**. Immunoglobulin A enters the cell after binding to its receptor, becomes internalized and is transported either to the Golgi apparatus or to the apical membrane of the cell for secretion. The third pathway involves the **synthesis and transport of milk lipids**. These lipids are synthesized in the cytoplasm and smooth endoplasmic reticulum after which they aggregate in droplets that coalesce to form larger fat globules that are discharged from the apical part of the cell into the alveolar lumen. The final pathway involves **exocytosis of secretory vesicles containing specific milk proteins, calcium, phosphate, citrate and lactose**. These vesicles form in the Golgi apparatus where casein, the specific milk protein, forms micelles with calcium and phosphate. The Golgi is impermeable to lactose, which is an osmotically active sugar so that water is drawn in. It is the lactose content that actually determines the liquid volume of the milk. A fifth pathway is not transcellular, but paracellular. Plasma proteins, immunoglobulins, especially IgA, and leukocytes can move between alveolar cells that have lost their tight junctions.

Regulation of milk production

The regulation of the quantity and content of breast milk is largely under hormonal control. The most important hormone in humans is **prolactin**, whose actions require synergism with several other hormones.

Prolactin concentrations in the plasma rise steadily throughout pregnancy from a baseline of less than 20 ng/mL to over 200 ng/mL at term (Chapter 17). In breast-feeding women, basal prolactin will remain elevated for about 4–6 weeks postpartum after which it falls to non-pregnant levels in spite of continued lactation. For about the next 2 months postpartum, suckling causes spikes of prolactin release; however, this reflex is gradually lost even with the production of a litre or more of breast milk per day.

The pivotal role of prolactin in the initiation of breast feeding was established by blocking the secretion of the hormone from the pituitary using the dopamine agonist, bromocriptine. When bromocriptine is given to women shortly after delivery, prolactin levels drop precipitously to non-pregnant levels. Breast engorgement and lactation never occur. Estrogens can also be used to suppress lactation immediately postpartum, but they work by a different mechanism. Prolactin levels remain quite elevated, but no milk is formed. Thus estrogens are inhibitory to the action of prolactin on the breast and are probably the reason why lactation does not occur before delivery. With delivery of the placenta, the source of the large amount of circulating estrogen is removed. Breast milk begins to form within 24–48 h after the circulating estrogens drop precipitously. Bromocriptine administered later in the postpartum period will inhibit lactation as long as it remains dependent on prolactin.

Prolactin has several actions at the cellular level. It stimulates the synthesis of both β-lactoglobulin and casein in breast tissue primed by insulin and cortisol. It also stabilizes casein mRNA, prolonging its half-life eight-fold, stimulates milk fat synthesis, and may be involved in sodium transport in mammary tissue. Interestingly, prolactin binding to its receptor does not stimulate adenylate cyclase activity as typically happens with other polypeptide hormones.

The lactation reflex

Although prolactin is responsible for the initiation of milk production, its delivery to the infant and the maintenance of lactation is dependent on mechanical stimulation of the nipple. The suckling stimulus is known as **milk ejection** or **letdown**. Although suckling is the major stimulus for milk letdown, the reflex can be conditioned. The cry or sight of an infant and preparation of the breast for nursing may cause letdown while pain, embarrassment and ethanol can inhibit it.

The suckling reflex is initiated when sensory impulses originating in the nipple enter the spinal cord through its dorsal roots. A multisynaptic neural pathway ascends to the magnocellular supraoptic and paraventricular nuclei of the hypothalamus via activin-containing neurons in the nucleus solitarius tract. Episodic **oxytocin** release from the posterior pituitary then occurs. The oxytocin stimulates the myoepithelial cells lining the milk ducts to contract, thereby causing milk 'ejection'.

Temporally associated with the episodic oxytocin release induced by nursing is a large surge of prolactin which is independent of the oxytocin. This transient pulse of prolactin induces milk formation for the next feeding. Smoking can inhibit this prolactin surge and cause a decrease in milk production.

The suckling reflex also affects the activity of the gonadotropin-releasing hormone (GnRH) pulse generator. Gonadotropin release is inhibited and ovulation does not occur. The effectiveness of lactation in suppressing gonadal function is directly related to the frequency and duration of nursing. Among the !Kung hunter-gatherers in Africa, the average interval between births is 44 months in spite of early postpartum resumption of coitus and lack of contraception. Mothers nurse about every 15 min and children are in immediate proximity to their mothers all day and night for 2 years or more.

21 Menopause

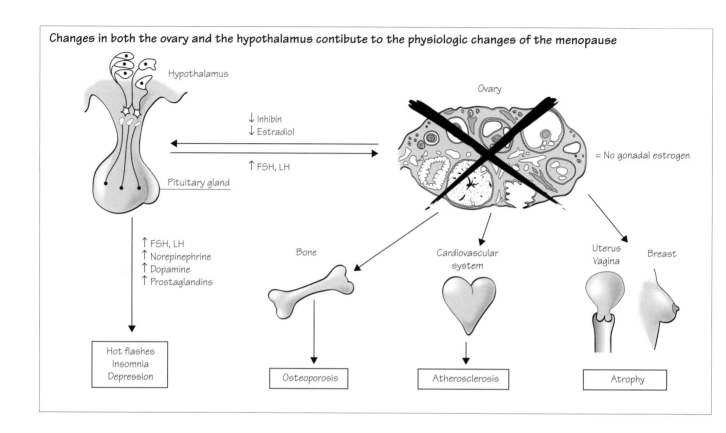

Changes in both the ovary and the hypothalamus contibute to the physiologic changes of the menopause

Hypothalamus

↓ Inhibin
↓ Estradiol

↑ FSH, LH

Pituitary gland

↑ FSH, LH
↑ Norepinephrine
↑ Dopamine
↑ Prostaglandins

Ovary

= No gonadal estrogen

Hot flashes
Insomnia
Depression

Bone

Cardiovascular
system

Uterus
Vagina

Breast

Osteoporosis

Atherosclerosis

Atrophy

Menopause is a normal stage of life with health consequences that have only become apparent as life expectancy has increased well beyond the 6th decade of life for women. It is estimated that women living in developed countries will live at least one-third of their lives after menopause. Functionally, menopause may be considered an **'estrogen withdrawal syndrome'**. It is recognizable by the universal loss of menses, typically in women in their late forties and early fifties, and for most women by the appearance of signs and symptoms such as hot flashes, insomnia, vaginal atrophy and decreased breast size and skin elasticity. The longer-term consequences of estrogen deficiency, osteoporosis and cardiovascular disease are both more indolent and less predictable than the early signs and symptoms of menopause.

Physiology of menopause

The postmenopausal ovary is small, shriveled and essentially devoid of follicles. The appearance of the postmenopausal ovary, coupled with the observation that oophorectomy is associated with menopausal symptoms, led to the original theory that follicular depletion was responsible for menopause. More recent evidence suggests that menopause has origins in both the central nervous system and ovary and that men also go through an andropause that is later and more subtle. The changes in the central nervous system and gonads that constitute 'gonopause' are now thought to be much more extensive and reflect aging in general.

Beginning at about age 40, fertility decreases dramatically in women. This fall in fertility is the first sign of impending ovarian fail-

ure. Although follicles remain visible on ultrasound, attempts at artificial induction of ovulation with injected gonadotropins are largely unsuccessful after about age 45 years. This suggests that a physiologic defect develops within the oocytes or follicles prior to their depletion. About 3–4 years before menopause is apparent, serum follicle-stimulating hormone (FSH) levels begin to rise subtly and ovarian estrogen, inhibin and progesterone production falls. Menstrual cycle length tends to decrease as the follicular phase shortens progressively and finally, ovulation and menstruation cease entirely. About one quarter of American women are menopausal by age 45 years; the mean age of menopause is 51 years of age in the United States.

Although ovarian failure is a major component of menopause, functional alterations occur at the level of the pituitary as well. The site of the change appears to be in the intrinsic rhythms, especially the circadian oscillator, which control sleep and the neuroendocrine axes. These changes lead to diminished nocturnal melatonin secretion and altered sleep, decreased responsiveness of the gonadotropin axis to steroid feedback and decreased adrenal steroid production. Aging is also associated with a more general decline in central dopaminergic and noradrenergic neuronal function; estrogen deficiency further exacerbates the dopamine deficiency by increasing the ratio of norepinephrine to dopamine.

During menopause, the decrease in ovarian estrogen and inhibin production leads to a progressive rise in gonadotropins because of the loss of normal negative feedback signals. FSH rises disproportionately to luteinizing hormone (LH) because of the loss of inhibin which acts exclusively to regulate FSH (Chapter 2). **When in doubt, persistent elevation of serum FSH levels confirms the diagnosis of menopause.** Although ovarian estrogen production essentially ceases, the ovary continues to make the androgens testosterone and androstenedione. Most of the steroid biosynthesis occurs in the hilar cells of the medulla of the gland and very little in the stroma. Hilar cells share a common embryologic origin with testicular Leydig cells, the main androgen-secreting cells in the male (Chapter 5.2).

Although ovarian estrogen production ceases at menopause, postmenopausal women are not totally estrogen deficient. Several peripheral tissues including fat, liver and kidney express the enzyme aromatase and can convert circulating androgens to estrogens. The major difference in peripheral conversion is that most of the estrogen produced is estrone. Estrone predominates because it is the estrogen produced from aromatization of androstenedione, the major androgen secreted by the postmenopausal ovary and adrenal gland (Chapter 3). Estrone is a very weak estrogen compared to estradiol. In the typical concentrations found in postmenopausal women, estrone does not provide protection against the long-term consequences of estrogen deficiency. A notable exception to this occurs in obese women. Fat is a particularly rich source of aromatase activity and obese postmenopausal women can produce substantial amounts of estrone. These high quantities of endogenous estrone provide some protection against the risk of menopausal vasomotor symptoms and osteoporosis but also expose the endometrium to unopposed estrogen stimulation. Prolonged exposure of the endometrium to estrogen without progesterone to convert it from a proliferative to secretory physiology places these women at increased risk of endometrial hyperplasia and carcinoma (Chapter 40). A similar risk of endometrial stimulation is present in women receiving estrogen alone for postmenopausal hormone replacement.

Signs and symptoms

Hot flashes

Hot flashes or flushes occur in about 75% of menopausal women. Nocturnal hot flashes are associated with waking and may produce significant sleep deprivation or insomnia. During a hot flash most women note a sensation of pressure in their head followed by a flush of heat or burning that begins on the head or neck area and passes over the entire body. Sweating invariably accompanies the flush. While there are profound physiologic changes that are associated with hot flashes, the mechanism by which estrogen deficiency produces this symptom is not known. The physiologic changes include an initial increase in skin conductance and then temperature, which reflects peripheral vasodilatation. Subsequently core body temperature drops by an average of 0.2°C. Circulating estrogens do not change before or after the flash but LH, cortisol, dehydroepiandrosterone (DHEA), androstenedione and the pro-opiomelanocortin (POM-C)-derived peptides all do. It is believed that the flash represents a change in central thermoregulation, which then elicits a number of compensatory mechanisms that transiently raise, but ultimately reduce the core temperature to the new set point. Central nervous system catecholamines are involved in hypothalamic temperature regulation and the impact of estrogen deficiency on noradrenergic neuronal function likely plays a role in hot flashes. One hypothesis is that estrogen deficiency predisposes to vasodilatation within the hypothalamus resulting in an increase in hypothalamic temperature.

In addition to hot flashes, most menopausal women experience **vaginal atrophy and changes in their breasts and skin**. Vaginal atrophy can lead to decreased lubrication and dyspareunia during intercourse. These changes are directly related to the loss of estrogen stimulation in target tissues and can largely be reversed by estrogen replacement.

Bone changes

Bone loss in women actually begins at about age 30 and accelerates at menopause. The most rapid bone loss occurs in the first 3–4 years after menopause and is accelerated in women who smoke and in very thin women. African-American race and fluoride treatment of the water supply are associated with a lower incidence of osteoporosis. The most common site of osteoporosis-related fractures is the vertebral body although the upper femur, humerus, ribs and distal forearm are also frequently affected. Upper femoral fractures that involve the hip joint may be life-threatening because of an accompanying risk of venous thromboembolic disease.

Osteoporosis resulting from prolonged estrogen deficiency involves a reduction in the quantity of bone without an alteration in its chemical composition. Bone formation by osteoblasts is normal but the rate of bone resorption by osteoclasts is increased. Trabecular bone is affected first, followed by cortical. Estrogen appears to antagonize the effects of parathyroid hormone (PTH) on calcium mobilization; estrogen receptors are found on bone cells in culture suggesting a direct effect of the hormone on bone.

Cardiovascular changes

Observational studies on the risk of **coronary artery disease** in postmenopausal women show a 40–50% reduction in incidence in women taking hormone replacement therapy. The only randomized, blinded controlled trial of hormone replacement therapy on cardiovascular risk was conducted in women who already had coronary artery disease. It showed an increased risk of venous thromboembolism early in the trial with no benefit by the end of the trial although an encouraging disease profile indicative of longer-term benefits was reported. In spite of the lack of prospective data on the effect of prophylactic estrogen replacement therapy on clinical coronary artery disease, the increase in high-density lipoproteins and decrease in low-density lipoproteins seen with hormone replacement therapy has been interpreted as a long-term benefit. Estrogen receptors are present on blood vessels and estrogen appears to clinically decrease vascular resistance and increase blood flow. One potential mechanism by which estrogen may improve blood flow is through its demonstrated ability to decrease the production of endothelin, a potent vasoconstrictor, by vascular endothelium.

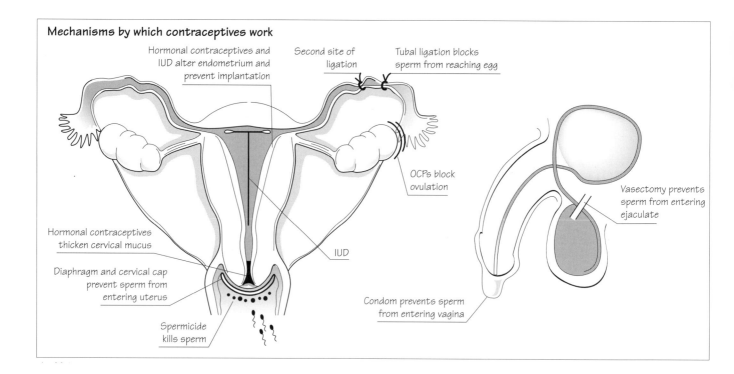

Mechanisms by which contraceptives work

Hormonal contraceptives and IUD alter endometrium and prevent implantation

Second site of ligation

Tubal ligation blocks sperm from reaching egg

OCPs block ovulation

Vasectomy prevents sperm from entering ejaculate

Hormonal contraceptives thicken cervical mucus

Diaphragm and cervical cap prevent sperm from entering uterus

IUD

Condom prevents sperm from entering vagina

Spermicide kills sperm

Overview

No form of contraception is perfect. Each has a finite failure rate that is linked both to the actual method itself and to the human frailties of the user. Most also have side-effects, some of which can be quite serious. The choice of the right contraceptive for an individual or a couple is a complex decision.

The risk of pregnancy in the absence of any contraception is 2–4% with each unprotected act of intercourse. This amounts to an overall pregnancy risk of 85 pregnancies per 100 woman years.

'Natural' family planning

The goal of natural family planning or fertility awareness is to abstain from intercourse during the woman's fertile period thereby avoiding conception. Natural family planning makes use of a calendar and some indicator of ovulation such as basal body temperature measurements, cervical mucus characteristics or commercial ovulation prediction kits to determine when a woman typically ovulates in her monthly menstrual cycle. Intercourse is then avoided during the so-called 'fertile period' and for several days before and after the fertile period. Use of natural family planning requires a highly motivated couple and the willingness to tolerate some risk of failure. It works best for women who have regular menstrual cycles.

Natural family planning has no medical side-effects and is accepted by virtually all religions. The failure rate of natural family planning varies between 5 and 35%, with most populations experiencing failure rates toward the higher figure.

Barrier methods

There are three general categories of barrier contraceptives: the condom, diaphragm and cervical cap. All three work by preventing spermatozoa from entering the woman's uterus and fertilizing an egg. Barrier methods are good for individuals who only want contraception when it is required and not all the time. The most serious side-effects of the barrier methods occur in individuals with an unknown latex allergy.

Condoms that fit over the man's penis are more widely available than female condoms which fit inside the woman's vagina. Male condoms may be made from latex rubber, polyurethane or animal intestines; each provides a different 'feel' or sensitivity for the man during intercourse. Female condoms are typically polyurethane. An intact condom prevents infectious agents as well as sperm from entering a woman's vagina and hence can prevent the transmission of HIV and other sexually transmitted diseases. A condom must be carefully removed after ejaculation so as to not spill the semen out into the vagina. Failure rates for condoms are 3–6% and may be improved by the use of a spermicide (see below).

The **diaphragm** is a soft latex or plastic dome that fits inside the vagina and covers the cervix. It is typically used together with a spermicide placed in the dome because some sperm may be able to bypass the diaphragm and gain access to the women's uterus. Diaphragms should be individually fitted by a health professional and some training is required in their proper insertion and removal. A diaphragm should be left in place for 6–8 h after intercourse; additional spermicide should be placed in the vagina if additional intercourse occurs before the diaphragm is removed. Diaphragms are partially protective against HIV and other sexually transmitted diseases. Some women develop bladder or vaginal infections from diaphragm use. The failure rate of a properly fitted diaphragm is about 6%; improper fitting or failure to use a spermicide increases the failure rate substantially.

Cervical caps are similar to the diaphragm except smaller. They fit tightly over the cervix and must be individually fitted in order to work at all. Cervical caps are not widely available.

Spermicides

Spermicides are chemicals that kill sperm by disrupting their outer cell membranes. The most commonly used spermicides are nonoxynol-9 and octoxynol-9. Spermicides are available suspended in one of three vehicles—foam, jelly or wax suppositories. They are maximally effective when used in conjunction with a barrier method. There are few absolute contraindications to use of a spermicide. They have an unpleasant taste and can cause an allergy in some users. The failure rate of spermicides used alone is 5–15%.

Intrauterine device

The **intrauterine device (IUD)** is a small T-shaped plastic device that is placed into the uterine cavity. It has a nylon thread attached which hangs down into the vagina so that the user can check that it remains in place. An IUD works by preventing implantation of the fertilized egg by several mechanisms. If the IUD is wrapped with copper, the mineral sets up a local inflammatory response in the endometrium which includes excess prostaglandin production. The copper ion competitively inhibits a number of zinc-requiring processes in the sperm and endometrium. If the IUD is impregnated with progestin, the normal proliferative–secretory sequence of endometrial maturation is disrupted, thereby making the intrauterine environment unsatisfactory for implantation.

IUDs have multiple medical contraindications because of their association with increased risk of sexually transmitted diseases. They are not recommended for women who have not had children nor those with multiple sexual partners. Significant side-effects include excessive menstrual bleeding, iron-deficiency anemia, dysmenorrhea and an increased risk for pelvic inflammatory disease (PID), infertility, ectopic pregnancy and septic abortion if pregnancy does occur. On the other hand, for a multiparous monogamous patient, the low failure rate (1–4%) and ease of use make it a very good contraceptive.

Hormonal contraception

Combination oral contraceptive pills (OCPs) are the most widely used form of hormonal contraception. They include a synthetic estrogen (ethinyl estradiol or mestranol) combined with a synthetic progestin (norethindrone, norgestrel or ethynodiol acetate) taken orally for 21 consecutive days of every 28. The estrogen and progestin dose may be constant over the 21 days or they may be sequential (phased or triphasic pills). Both types of combination OCPs prevent pregnancy by multiple mechanisms including inhibition of ovulation, thickening of cervical mucus so that sperm cannot readily penetrate it and alteration of the uterine lining to block implantation.

OCPs appear to have some health benefits beyond pregnancy prevention. These include decreased risks for PID, benign breast disease, anemia and endometrial and ovarian cancer. They are not totally risk free, however, and are associated with increased risk of thromboembolic disease and gallbladder disease. Women over the age of 35 years who smoke should not use OCPs. Failure rates for OCPs are 0.5–2%. In order to be effective, OCPs must be taken in the correct order on a daily basis.

Progestin-only contraceptives are effective by both the oral and parenteral route. They all work by thickening cervical mucus and altering the endometrial lining of the uterus, thereby preventing sperm from reaching the site of fertilization and any eggs that may fertilize from implanting. In some women, progestin alone will also prevent ovulation. The oral form of the progestin-only contraceptive is known as the 'mini-pill' and is useful in women who have contraindications to estrogen such as breast feeding. The mini-pill has a failure rate of 1–3%.

Depo-Provera is the injectable form of progestin. It is given as an intramuscular injection every 90 days. Norplant is a system of six soft capsules of progestin which are implanted under the skin. They may be left in place for 5 years. The advantage of the parenteral forms of hormonal contraception is that, once they are in place, they require no effort on the part of the woman. The disadvantage is that they are not readily reversible, as one must wait for Depo-Provera to clear the system or surgically remove the Norplant in cases of serious side-effects or a desire for pregnancy. The failure rate for Depo-Provera is 1% and between 0.2% and 1.6% for Norplant.

Emergency hormonal contraception ('morning-after pill') can be effective in preventing pregnancy if taken within 72 h of unprotected intercourse or a contraceptive failure. The morning-after pill uses the same hormones as found in combination OCPs only in higher doses. The mechanisms by which pregnancy can be prevented are the same three that occur with combination OCPs.

Sterilization

Sterilization of both men and women are surgical methods of permanent contraception. Sterilization prevents the gametes from reaching the point of fertilization. In women, surgical options consist of tubal ligation and hysterectomy. Tubal ligation involves surgical interruption of the Fallopian tubes with cautery, incision or banding so that sperm can no longer reach the egg to fertilize it. Tubal ligations have a low failure rate (0–1%) depending on the exact surgical technique used. If a pregnancy does occur following tubal ligation, it has a 40–50% chance of implantation in an ectopic (tubal) location because of the blockage of the Fallopian tube entrance into the uterus. Hysterectomies are rarely performed solely for sterilization but do eliminate the possibility of pregnancy.

The sterilization procedure in men is called a **vasectomy**. It involves cutting and tying or cauterizing the ends of the vas deferens as they leave the testes in the scrotum. Vasectomy is 100% effective after a waiting period of 3 months. Vasectomy is a risk factor for prostate cancer (Chapter 38).

23 Common mechanisms in endocrine disorders

Mechanisms by which endocrine disorders develop.

	↓ Or absent hormone activity		↑ Hormone activity	
	↓ Hormone	↓ Receptor	↑ Hormone	↑ Receptor
Genetic	Enzyme block Mutant hormone Absent trophic signal	Mutant receptor	Upstream from enzyme block Decreased degradation	Mutant receptor
Acquired	Autoimmune destruction of endocrine gland Drugs Loss of trophic signal Surgical removal of endocrine gland	Autoimmune destruction of target gland Blocking antibodies Drugs Surgical removal of target gland	Stimulating autoantibodies ↑ Production Drugs	Stimulating autoantibodies Drugs
Neoplastic	Replacement of endocrine gland with tumor	Replacement of target tissue with tumor	↑ Trophic hormone Autonomous hormone production	Somatic cell mutations

All endocrine disorders are ultimately the result of too little or too much hormone activity at a target site. There are, however, multiple ways in which the abnormal activity may develop. The following is an overview of the ways in which endocrine disorders can arise, especially those that can affect the reproductive system.

Genetic mutations

Mutations can occur in genes responsible for any step in a hormone's action, from its synthesis to its interaction with a receptor to its degradation. These mutations can affect the entire organism (germ-line mutations) or specific tissues (somatic cell mutations). **Germ-line mutations** are gene mutations present in one or both parents that are transmitted via the sperm and/or egg to their offspring. Examples of endocrine disorders transmitted as germ-line mutations include congenital adrenal hyperplasia and pseudovaginal perineoscrotal hypospadias. These disorders are two of the more commonly encountered **autosomal recessive disorders** affecting the reproductive system. Congenital adrenal hyperplasia develops when each parent has one abnormal gene for the same enzyme in the steroid biosynthetic pathway and the fetus inherits both defective genes. The fetus is then exposed to abnormally high concentrations of androgen precursors upstream from the enzyme block. Female fetuses are born with masculinized or ambiguous genitalia (Chapter 25). Pseudovaginal perineoscrotal hypospadias is caused by a deficiency in the enzyme 5α-reductase. Males who inherit two copies of the mutant gene are born with a female phenotype but masculinize at puberty (Chapter 24).

Androgen receptor abnormalities are **sex-linked** because the gene for the androgen receptor is on the X chromosome. Unaffected carrier females will have a mutation in the androgen receptor on one of their two X chromosomes. This abnormality is silent because of the normal androgen receptor gene on the other X. Males who inherit the affected X chromosome from their mothers have only the one defective androgen receptor gene and display the syndrome of androgen insensitivity (Chapter 24). Many different mutations of the androgen receptor have been reported in affected families. Each alters receptor function in a unique way, producing different phenotypes ranging from complete androgen insensitivity to isolated azoospermia.

Somatic cell mutations are typically sporadic and produce different diseases depending on when and where in development the mutation occurs. For example, mutations that occur early in fetal life will produce syndromes with protean manifestations because of the multitude of affected cells. Mutations that occur late in fetal life or after birth produce phenotypes that may be restricted to one or a few organs depending on the exact location and timing. An example of a disorder produced by a somatic cell mutation is the McCune–Albright syndrome. McCune–Albright syndrome is defined as the constellation of café-au-lait spots, polyostotic fibrous dysplasia and gonadotropin-releasing hormone (GnRH)-independent sexual precocity. It results from a mutation in the gene for a G protein. This in turn produces hyperstimulation of the cAMP pathway in the affected tissues. McCune–Albright syndrome develops only if the somatic cell mutation occurs in late fetal life; earlier mutations cause multiple endocrinopathies (growth hormone (GH)-secreting pituitary adenomas, hyperthyroidism, autonomous adrenal hyperfunction) in addition to the precocious puberty. Somatic cell G-protein mutations in the adult cause isolated neoplasms such as pituitary or thyroid adenomas.

Acquired endocrinopathies

There are many reasons for acquired abnormalities in endocrine function. These include stimulation or destruction of a gland by autoantibodies or infectious agents, acquisition of hormone resistance, medication use, compression of an endocrine gland by a nearby mass and surgical removal of an endocrine gland.

Autoimmune destruction of glandular tissue is one of the most common causes of endocrine hypofunction. Type I diabetes mellitus, primary hypothyroidism and premature ovarian failure are all disorders caused by autoantibodies that destroy the hormone-producing cells of an endocrine gland. Autoimmune destruction of the ovaries is the leading non-surgical cause of premature menopause.

Graves' disease is an example of **autoimmune hyperstimulation** of the thyroid gland; viral infections also can cause transient syndromes of thyroid hormone excess. Once an individual has begun making auto-antibodies against one endocrine organ, he or she is at increased risk of developing antibodies against another gland. At least 30% of individuals with an autoimmune endocrine disorder will demonstrate autoantibodies against another gland. Many of the women with premature ovarian failure have either overt or covert evidence of autoimmune thyroiditis or autoantibodies against intrinsic factor (pernicious anemia).

Interestingly, women are much more prone to develop autoimmune disorders, outnumbering men 6 : 1 in prevalence. The reason for this large gender difference is unknown, but is thought to involve the influence of ovarian estrogens. This theory has arisen because infants, children and older adults only show a female : male ratio of 2 : 1 and because many women with systemic lupus erythematosus demonstrate unusually high concentrations of urinary estrogens.

Resistance syndromes occur in individuals who have inherited a cellular abnormality in the ability of a target organ to respond to a particular hormone and who then lose their ability to produce adequate amounts of hormone to overcome the defect. The cellular defects commonly encountered include abnormal receptors for the hormone, defects in the metabolism of the hormone or defects in the intracellular signaling pathways necessary for the hormone to exert its action. The best known resistance syndrome is type II diabetes. In type II diabetes the abnormalities in insulin receptor action are initially overcome by oversecreting insulin. Hyperglycemia does not develop until the pancreas is unable to secrete sufficient insulin to overcome the receptor defect. Obesity plays a major role in the development of type II diabetes in most patients through an unknown mechanism. **Defective function of the insulin receptor and insulin resistance are commonly found in the subset of women with polycystic ovary syndrome (PCOS) who are obese.** Treatment with insulin sensitizing agents treats both their type II diabetes and their PCOS. Some non-obese women with PCOS appear to have abnormal responses to either growth hormone or gonadotropins.

In addition to unmasking resistance syndromes, **obesity** can also cause endocrinopathies directly. Adipocytes contain both aromatase and 17-hydroxysteroid dehydrogenase, two enzymes important in the conversion of androgens to estrogens. Obese postmenopausal women, especially those with obesity of the lower body, can produce large amounts of estrogens by converting adrenal androstenedione to estrone in their adipocytes. Obesity is also associated with a decrease in estrogen degradation, thereby further enhancing the hyperestrogenic state.

Medications that block the interaction of a hormone with its receptor or inhibit its biosynthesis are purposely used to treat endocrinopathies; however, medications commonly used to treat non-endocrine disorders may also lead to endocrinopathies. For example, the estrogen agonist/antagonist tamoxifen is used in the treatment of breast cancer. In the breast, tamoxifen acts as an antiestrogen whereas the estrogen receptors in the endometrium are stimulated by the drug. Cimetidine, the H_2-blocker originally developed to treat peptic ulcer disease, has a mild stimulatory effect at the androgen receptor. Older antidepressants and other centrally active medications with antidopaminergic activity can cause hyperprolactinemia and amenorrhea.

The most common gland affected by compression from a nearby mass is the pituitary. The susceptibility of the pituitary to mass effects stems both from its location in the limited space within the sella turcica and from the exposed neuroendocrine and vascular connections to it that travel through the median eminence. Surgery to remove suprachiasmatic masses such as craniopharyngiomas or teratomas may also secondarily cause hypopituitarism because of the difficulty in removing the tumor without disrupting the sella or the tissue connections to the pituitary. Surgical extirpation of the pituitary, ovaries or testes will produce endocrinopathies if removal of the gland is complete.

Neoplastic endocrinopathies

Somatic cell mutations can result in specific reproductive tract neoplasms with endocrine consequences (Chapters 35–41). These can occur either sporadically or in individuals who have inherited germ-line mutations in tumor suppressor genes or proto-oncogenes. Families who carry mutations in the retinoblastoma (RET) proto-oncogene are at increased risk for the multiple endocrine neoplasia 2 syndromes which include medullary carcinoma of the thyroid, pheochromocytomas and hyperparathyroidism. Sporadically occurring reproductive tract neoplasms that overproduce hormones are the Leydig and Sertoli cell tumors of the gonads which secrete enormous amounts of androgen and estrogen, respectively (Chapters 37 and 39).

Some endocrinopathies may, in fact, contribute to neoplasia. For example, continuous stimulation of the endometrium by estrogen, such as occurs in PCOS or in obese postmenopausal women, can contribute to the development of endometrial carcinoma (Chapter 40). Androgen excess appears to be a risk factor for developing prostate cancer. Androgen antagonism or withdrawal is a mainstay in its treatment (Chapter 38).

Conversely, some inherited or somatic cell endocrine mutations are protective against neoplasia. Men who lack the enzyme 5α-reductase, which converts testosterone to dihydrotestosterone, do not develop prostate glands and are not at risk for prostatic neoplasms (Chapter 38).

24 Abnormalities of male sexual differentiation and development

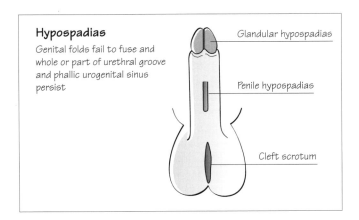

Hypospadias

Genital folds fail to fuse and whole or part of urethral groove and phallic urogenital sinus persist

- Glandular hypospadias
- Penile hypospadias
- Cleft scrotum

Cryptorchidism

An undescended testis (cryptorchidism) is the most common genital abnormality seen in male newborns. It occurs in 3% of newborns. Either one or both testes may be involved. Cryptorchidism occurs when the gubernaculum fails either to develop or to pull the testes into the scrotum. All evidence points to a failure of androgen activity on the gubernaculum as the etiology for the disorder. The lack of androgen activity can result from developmental defects anywhere along the fetal hypothalamic–pituitary–testicular axis. Thus fetal hypothalamic failure to stimulate gonadotropin secretion in the third trimester (Kallman and Prader–Willi syndromes, anencephaly), failure of the testes to secrete androgens (gonadal dysgenesis), failure of testosterone conversion to dihydrotestosterone in target tissues (5α-reductase deficiency) or absence of functioning androgen receptors (androgen insensitivity syndromes) can lead to cryptorchidism. Interestingly, the mothers of cryptorchid newborns have later menarche and shorter menses, suggesting a role for subtle maternal hypogonadism or an inherited tendency toward the same in the development of cryptorchidism. *In utero* diethylstilbestrol (DES) exposure is associated with an increased incidence of cryptorchidism, again suggesting that maternal estrogen abnormalities are involved in the development of the disorder.

The testes may remain in the inguinal canal (70%), the abdomen or retroperitoneum (25%), or other ectopic locations (5%). Testes remaining in the abdomen or inguinal canal will become incapable of normal spermatogenesis because of the higher temperatures there when compared to the scrotum. They are also prone to developing cancer. Therapy for cryptorchidism is either medical using human chorionic gonadotropin (hCG) or androgen administration or surgical (orchiopexy). Cryptorchid testes that cannot be brought into the scrotum are usually removed because they cannot be adequately watched for the development of a neoplasm.

Inguinal hernia is a forme fruste of cryptorchidism in which testicular descent occurs, but the inguinal ring does not close completely. Boys who have inguinal hernia diagnosed before the age of 15 have twice the risk of developing testicular cancer than the general population.

Hypospadias

Another very common congenital abnormality seen in male newborns is hypospadias. In hypospadias, the urethral meatus opens onto the ventral surface of the penile shaft proximal to the normal location. Embryologically, hypospadias occurs when the urethral groove fails to close completely. Because the penile urethra depends on the androgen dihydrotestosterone (DHT) to differentiate, hypospadias can result from either a deficiency in testosterone (T) production, inadequate conversion of T to DHT, or a local deficiency in androgen receptors. There is a non-Mendelian genetic predisposition to hypospadias. If one sibling has a hypospadias, the recurrence risk is 12%. If both the father and a brother are affected, the risk for a second son is 25%.

Cryptorchidism is seen in 16% of boys with hypospadias. If both are present, the child may be a pseudohermaphrodite (see below) and a karyotype and hormonal testing should be obtained.

Congenital bilateral absence of the vas deferens

Congenital bilateral absence of the vas deferens (CBAVD) is a rare congenital anomaly usually seen in men with cystic fibrosis (CF). It can also occur in the absence of clinically apparent CF. When it does, it is usually associated with mutations in the gene coding for the CF transmembrane receptor (CFTR). The molecular mechanism by which an abnormal transmembrane receptor involved in chloride channels leads either to failure of the vas deferens to differentiate or to its resorption is not known. CBAVD is an indication for genetic testing for CF genes.

Pseudohermaphroditism

Male pseudohermaphroditism occurs when testes are present but the external, and sometimes internal, genitalia have a female phenotype. Male pseudohermaphroditism results from an inappropriate fetal hormonal environment caused either by a biochemical defect in androgen activity or by an abnormal sex chromosome constitution. Pseudohermaphroditism is a rare disorder, but its multiple etiologies have offered the opportunity to further understand the role of steroids in human genital development. A list of the known biochemical defects leading to male pseudohermaphroditism includes:

- Androgen insensitivity syndromes.
- 5α-Reductase deficiency.
- Testosterone biosynthesis defects.
- Lipoid congenital adrenal hyperplasia (StAR protein deficiency).
- 3β-Hydroxysteroid dehydrogenase deficiency.
- 17α-Hydroxylase deficiency.
- 17β-Hydroxysteroid dehydrogenase deficiency.
- Impaired androgenization.
- Anti-Müllerian hormone defect.

Androgen insensitivity syndromes

The androgen insensitivity syndromes are a group of X-linked recessive traits that produce a spectrum of incompletely virilized phenotypes. The most severe form, **complete androgen insensitivity (AI)**, was originally known as **testicular feminization**. In complete AI, the intracellular androgen receptor is either absent or non-functional. Androgen induction of Wolffian duct development does not occur.

Müllerian-inhibiting substance (MIS) is produced by the testes, however, and the Müllerian ducts regress. The testes descend to the level of the inguinal ring under the influence of MIS. A short vagina forms from the urogenital sinus. At birth, these children are assigned the female sex because there is no trace of androgen activity and the external genitalia are clearly female. Complete AI is typically diagnosed after puberty when primary amenorrhea becomes apparent. Examination of the complete AI individual reveals a blind-ending, short vagina and an absent cervix, uterus and ovaries. Breast development is normal, but axillary and pubic hair is scant or absent. Complete AI accounts for about 10% of all cases of primary amenorrhea. In contrast to those individuals with a dysgenetic gonad bearing a Y chromosome (see below), those with complete AI have less than a 5% risk of developing a gonadal tumor and the tumors rarely appear before age 25. Therefore, gonadectomy is postponed until puberty is complete.

The **incomplete androgen insensitivity syndrome (Reifenstein syndrome)** is far less common than the complete and is associated with a broad spectrum of phenotypes that varies from almost complete failure of virilization to essentially complete phenotypic masculinization. Between these extremes exist patients with mild clitoromegaly and slight labial fusion to those with significant genital ambiguity. Recently, several men have been described whose only indication of AI was infertility because of low or absent sperm. Some fertile males who appear undervirilized probably have a mild form of this disorder.

Incomplete AI results from mutations in the androgen receptor gene. The gene encoding the androgen receptor localizes to the q11–12 region of the X chromosome. Defects occur in both the androgen binding domain and the DNA binding domain as well as in receptor protein production. The abnormalities identified range from complete loss of receptor function to subtle qualitative changes in the stimulation and transcription of androgen dependent target genes. There is not a good correlation between receptor levels, hence quantitative androgen binding, and the degree of masculinization seen in incomplete AI.

5α-Reductase deficiency
The syndrome seen with 5α-reductase deficiency was originally given the name **pseudovaginal perineoscrotal hypospadias (PPH)**. It differs from AI in that masculinization occurs at puberty. At birth, individuals with 5α-reductase deficiency have external genitalia that resemble those of incomplete AI, including hypospadias, varying degrees of failure of the labioscrotal folds to fuse and either a urogenital opening or separate vaginal and urethral openings. The cleft in the scrotum resembles a vagina and hence, most of these children are raised as girls. Adrenal steroid production is normal and the karyotype is XY, eliminating the possibility of congenital adrenal hyperplasia in a female newborn as a cause for the incomplete virilization (Chapter 25). Measuring the blood levels of testosterone and dihydrotestosterone and demonstrating an elevated T : DHT ratio can establish the diagnosis.

Molecular analyses have demonstrated that there are two 5α-reductase genes; mutations in the isoenzyme coded on chromosome 2 (*SRD5A2* gene) are responsible for this form of male pseudohermaphroditism. Multiple mutations of *SRD5A2* have been identified. The segregation of the same specific defects in unrelated individuals of the same ethnicity suggests a degree of common ancestry. Women are not clinically affected by 5α-reductase deficiency and compound heterozygotes are common, suggesting that the gene frequency for *SRD5A2* mutations may be fairly high.

Congenital adrenal hyperplasia syndromes
Lipoid congenital adrenal hyperplasia (StAR protein deficiency), 3β-hydroxysteroid dehydrogenase deficiency, 17α-hydroxylase deficiency and 17β-hydroxysteroid dehydrogenase deficiency are all specific enzymatic defects in the steroidogenic pathway common to the testes and adrenal glands. Together with several other enzymatic defects of the steroidogenic pathways, these defects are collectively known as the congenital adrenal hyperplasia (CAH) syndromes. The CAH syndromes that result in feminization of the fetal external genitalia all involve enzymes occurring early in the steroidogenic pathway between cholesterol and testosterone (Chapters 3 and 27).

Gender assignment
Gender assignment in male infants with pseudohermaphroditism requires knowledge of the specific defect. Most are raised as females. Individuals with complete AI (testicular feminization) are raised as females because they appear unambiguously as females at birth and they cannot be virilized at all, due to the lack of functional androgen receptors. Males whose incomplete AI presents with ambiguous genitalia usually are raised as females because of the feminization with gynecomastia that will occur at puberty. Males with 5α-reductase deficiency have been successfully raised either as females or as males, and in some cultures with a high frequency of the disorder, as females in childhood and males after puberty. Patients assigned as females who wish to retain their female gender will need to be gonadectomized to avoid deepening of their voices and a male pattern of muscle development under the influence of testosterone, to which they can respond. Estrogen and progesterone therapy will produce female secondary sexual development. Patients assigned to the male gender require repair of their hypospadias and cryptorchidism. At puberty, spermatogenesis and masculine sexual maturation will occur under the influence of testosterone.

True gonadal dysgenesis is relatively rare in individuals with an XY karyotype. Bilateral dysgenesis of the testes (**Swyer syndrome**) results in normal, but infantile female external and internal genitalia and lack of secondary sexual development at puberty. Fibrous bands appear in place of the testes. Gonadectomy is necessary to prevent the 20–30% risk of tumor formation. Estrogen and progesterone therapy supports female secondary sexual development at puberty.

The androgen insensitivity syndromes.

	Complete	Reifenstein	Infertile	5α-Reductase
Inheritance	X-linked recessive	X-linked recessive	X-linked recessive	Autosomal recessive
Spermatogenesis	Absent	Absent	Decreased	Decreased
Müllerian structures	Absent	Absent	Absent	Absent
Wolffian structures	Absent	Male	Male	Male
External genitalia	Female	Male/hypospadias	Male	Female
Breasts (puberty)	Female	Female/gynecomastia	Gynecomastia	Male

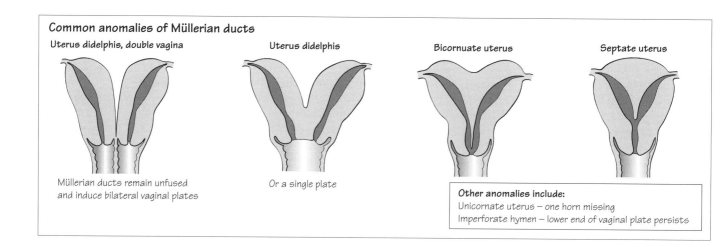

Common anomalies of Müllerian ducts

Uterus didelphis, double vagina

Müllerian ducts remain unfused and induce bilateral vaginal plates

Uterus didelphis

Or a single plate

Bicornuate uterus

Septate uterus

Other anomalies include:
Unicornate uterus – one horn missing
Imperforate hymen – lower end of vaginal plate persists

Structural anomalies

Structural anomalies of the uterus, cervix and vagina are the most common abnormalities of sexual differentiation seen in women. They arise from embryologic abnormalities of the Müllerian system (Chapter 5.3). The most severe form involves complete absence of the reproductive tract including the vagina, uterus and Fallopian tubes. This disorder, which arises from agenesis of the Müllerian system, is known as Mayer–Rokitansky–Kuster–Hauser syndrome. This syndrome is the second most common cause of primary amenorrhea (see Chapter 28).

The remainder of the anomalies result from failure of the Müllerian system either to fuse or to remodel in the midline to form a single uterine cavity. The most dramatic form of fusion anomaly occurs when the Müllerian ducts fail to fuse along their entire length, resulting in the formation of two vaginas, two cervices and two separate uterine horns (double uterus or *uterus didelphis*). More commonly only the upper portion of the uterus is separated as two horns (bicornuate uterus or *uterus bicornus*) or a dimple remains in the uterine fundus (arcuate uterus). Occasionally, only one side of the Müllerian system will develop resulting in hemi-uterus and single Fallopian tube (unicornuate uterus or *uterus unicornus*).

Failure of resorption of the midline of the Müllerian ducts after fusion occurs typically results in a uterine septum. A septum may be complete, running from the cervix to the fundus, or incomplete, involving only the uterine fundus (subseptate uterus). Occasionally the vagina will not canalize properly and a vaginal septum will occur, either alone or in conjunction with a uterine anomaly. Vaginal septa can be either longitudinal or horizontal. The longitudinal septum is reminiscent of the uterine anomalies resulting from failure of the Müllerian midline to resorb whereas the horizontal septa are thought to represent failure of the vaginal plate to resorb at the site where the Müllerian ducts fuse with it. Although the exact mechanism by which these anomalies form is not known, most anomalies seem to represent various degrees of failure of the Müllerian ducts to fuse or to remodel in the midline.

Although many women with structural anomalies are asymptomatic and never diagnosed, these Müllerian tract abnormalities can be associated with primary amenorrhea, recurrent miscarriages, preterm delivery and breech presentation at term. **Because of the involvement of the mesonephros in directing the development of the internal genitalia, the finding of a uterine anomaly should prompt an evaluation of the urinary system for an accompanying renal or ureteral anomaly.**

Exposure to diethylstilbestrol

In utero exposure to diethylstilbestrol (DES) occurred in individuals born between 1940 and 1972 whose mothers were given the synthetic estrogen in the hope of preventing a miscarriage. DES was subsequently shown to cause congenital abnormalities in women and, to a lesser degree, in men. The most frequently seen abnormalities in women are abnormally shaped cervices described as either coxcomb, hooded or hypoplastic. The uterine musculature may also be abnormally formed such that the cavity assumes a 'T' shape on hysterosalpingography. *In utero* DES exposure is associated with an increased risk of reproductive failure largely from preterm delivery. The mechanism by which DES appears to have caused the abnormalities is inappropriate activation of estrogen-dependent genes involved in differentiating the cervix and upper third of the vagina from the lower vagina. This results not only in the structurally abnormal cervices and uteri, but also in persistence of cervical glandular epithelium in the vagina (**vaginal adenosis**). DES daughters are at increased risk for malignancies arising in the vaginal adenosis because it is exposed to inducers not usually accessible to the upper reproductive tract.

While it can be surmised from animal experiments that timing of the DES exposure is critical to determining the degree of abnormality, it is rarely possible to determine when a given woman was exposed. This is largely related to inadequate medical documentation from decades ago. Occasionally, clinicians will observe cervical and uterine abnormalities that look exactly like those caused by *in utero* DES exposure in the documented absence of exposure to DES.

Congenital adrenal hyperplasia

Ambiguous genitalia in a newborn infant are most commonly caused by congenital adrenal hyperplasia (CAH). This diagnosis accounts for

40–50% of all cases of ambiguous genitalia. Affected female infants have perineal structures that include a common urogenital sinus containing the vagina and urethra, which opens at the base of an enlarged phallus resembling a penis. The labia majora may be hypertrophied or fused and thus resemble an empty scrotum. The infant typically looks like a male with hypospadias and cryptorchidism. While some of these infants will have hypertension (5%) or life-threatening salt wasting (30%) to aid in the differential diagnosis, those carrying the most common defect, moderate 21β-hydroxylase deficiency, will have no other identifying findings. **The finding of a normal female karyotype in a newborn assigned to the male gender in the delivery room requires an evaluation for CAH.**

The primary defect in all types of CAH is the absence of one of the enzymes necessary for steroidogenesis. The most common forms involve the enzymes that convert androgens to the adrenal steroids (see table below). In the absence of the enzyme, no end product will be produced to feed back on the hypothalamic–pituitary axis to regulate ACTH secretion. Excess ACTH will continue to stimulate the adrenals to produce more steroid precursors. Adrenal hyperplasia with excess androgen production will result. This is of no consequence in the male fetus but will result in masculinization of the androgen-sensitive external genitalia in a female. Because there are no testes and hence no Müllerian-inhibiting substance, females affected by CAH will have uteri and vaginas. The degree of hypertrophy and fusion of the external genitalia is dependent on the timing in development of the androgen effect and the quantity of androgen involved.

Therapy for these **masculinized female infants** (female pseudo-hermaphrodites) with CAH is both administration of glucocorticoid to suppress androgen secretion by the adrenals and reconstructive surgery. Infants who also have a defect in aldosterone synthesis need mineralocorticoid replacement as well.

Virilization of female infants occurs only when androgens are unable to be converted to estrogens by placental aromatase. Therefore, infants born to mothers with CAH are not at risk unles the child has inherited the genetic defect from both parents. Infants born to mothers with an androgen-producing tumor may be virilized if the androgen produced cannot be aromatized (e.g. dihydrotestosterone, DHT) or it quantitatively exceeds the high capacity of the placenta. Maternal administration of synthetic progestins with androgenic activity has also been associated with virilization of the female neonate, so use of synthetic progesterones is contraindicated in pregnant women. Female virilization that resulted from steroid exposure *in utero* with no risk of postnatal exposure is treated with reconstructive surgery alone.

Turner syndrome

Women with Turner syndrome are usually identifiable because of the associated physical characteristics of short stature, webbed neck, shield chest and increased carrying angle accompanying primary amenorrhea. The fundamental defect in Turner syndrome is absence of a second sex chromosome, i.e. a 45X karyotype. In the absence of a functional second sex chromosome, the germ cells in the gonad do not survive the embryonic period and a normal ovary or testis does not develop. Gonadal steroid synthesis and secretion do not occur either during embryogenesis or at puberty. Turner syndrome is the most common of a group of disorders known as **gonadal dysgenesis**.

The phenotype of most individuals with gonadal dysgenesis is female at birth. If all of the second sex chromosome is missing, both the external and internal genitalia will be female. After puberty, these female structures will remain infantile because of the lack of ovarian estrogens from the non-functional gonad. If there is any remnant of either sex chromosome present, the phenotype will depend on the specific genes retained. For instance, if the SRY locus is translocated onto another chromosome, the signal to begin testicular differentiation will occur. Müllerian-inhibiting substance (MIS) will be made and the Müllerian duct system will essentially disappear. These individuals will be born with female external genitalia due to a lack of androgen production by the rudimentary testis but will lack a vagina, uterus and Fallopian tubes. Primordial Wolffian ducts may be identified at laparotomy along with ovotestes. These rare individuals are true hermaphrodites.

Sex chromosome **mosaicism** (multiple cell lines of different chromosome composition) is not uncommon in Turner syndrome. Individuals carrying any portion of the Y chromosome, including SRY alone, may have a testicular component to their dysgenetic gonad. These patients are at risk for both virilization at puberty from functional testicular tissue and for gonadal malignancies. Therefore it is important to confirm a suspected diagnosis of Turner syndrome by karyotype (some experts recommend using a DNA probe against SRY as well). Individuals who have a cell line containing a Y chromosome or who carry SRY should have a bilateral gonadectomy prior to puberty to eliminate the possibility of virilization or cancer.

If the mosaicism involves a second X chromosome, functional ovarian tissue can be anticipated to exist within the gonad. These women may experience normal female puberty and even be fertile for a brief period of time. Early menopause occurs because of the limited number of functional follicles resulting from the abnormal chromosomal constitution. A woman with complete Turner syndrome or XX mosaicism can carry a pregnancy conceived through *in vitro* fertilization using donated oocytes and hormonal priming of her infantile uterus.

'Virilizing' forms of congenital adrenal hyperplasia.

Enzyme deficiency	Clinical appearance	Cortisol	Aldosterone	Androgens
21β-Hydroxylase—severe	Salt-wasting, virilized	–	–	++
21β-Hydroxylase—moderate	Virilized	Normal	+	++
21β-Hydroxylase—mild	Adult polycystic ovaries	Normal	+/–	+
11β-Hydroxylase	Hypertensive, virilized	–	–	++
17α-Hydroxylase	Hypertensive	–	+/–	–

26 Precocious puberty

Classification of precocious puberty.

Complete isosexual precocity (true precocious puberty—gonadotropin dependent)
Idiopathic
CNS lesions
   Hamartomas
   Craniopharyngioma
Primary hypothyroidism
Following treatment for virilizing disorders in girls

Incomplete isosexual precocity (GnRH independent)
Estrogen-secreting neoplasms of ovary or adrenal in girls
Ovarian cysts
Androgen-secreting neoplasms of testis or adrenal in boys
McCune–Albright syndrome
Peutz–Jeghers syndrome

Iatrogenic sexual precocity

Contrasexual precocity
Virilization in females
   Congenital adrenal hyperplasia
   21-Hydroxylase deficiency
   11β-Hydroxylase deficiency
   3β-Hydroxysteroid dehydrogenase deficiency
   Androgen-secreting ovarian or adrenal neoplasms
Feminization in males
   Estrogen-secreting adrenal neoplasms

Sexual precocity is defined as the appearance of secondary sexual characteristics before the age of 8 years in girls and 9 years in boys. Although recent data suggest that these ages are less than two standard deviations from the mean, breast or pubic hair development before age 8 or menarche before age 10 warrants an evaluation in girls, as does testicular enlargement or pubic hair development before age 9 in boys. While the appearance of all secondary sex characteristics results from increased sex steroid production, the cause of the increase may be increased gonadotropin secretion or intrinsic disease of the adrenal, ovary or testes. **Complete or true sexual precocity** is used to describe precocious puberty resulting from elevated pituitary gonadotropins. **Incomplete or peripheral sexual precocity** refers to precocious puberty resulting from primary diseases of the gonads or adrenals. Early sexual development that is consistent with the sex of the individual is **isosexual precocity**. **Heterosexual** or **contrasexual precocity** indicates precocious puberty associated with feminization of a male or virilization of a female.

Although over half of the cases of isosexual precocious puberty simply represent the early end of the normal developmental spectrum, it is important to evaluate all children with sexual precocity for several reasons. First, the child may be suffering from a serious disorder associated with precocious puberty. Second, if left untreated, sexual precocity occuring before age 6–7 years can be associated with short stature in adulthood. Finally, **sexual precocity is not accompanied by advanced psychosexual maturation**. Unfortunately young girls with precocious puberty appear to be at significant risk for sexual abuse.

Ovulation and conception are possible; pregnancies in girls as young as 5 years of age have occured as the result of such abuse. Appropriate therapy and support are necessary to prevent the potential long-term consequences of sexual precocity.

True or complete precocious puberty

True sexual precocity results from early maturation of the hypothalamic–pituitary–gonadal axis. Serum gonadotropins and sex steroid concentrations are in the normal postpubertal range as is gonadotropin pulsatility. The physical characteristics of puberty appear in the proper chronological order, just too early.

Central nervous system (CNS) lesions account for the other half of the cases of complete isosexual precocity. These lesions include neoplasms, trauma, hydrocephalus, postinfectious encephalitis, congenital brain defects, tuberous sclerosis and neurofibromatosis type I. Typically, the lesions are located in, or near, the posterior hypothalamus. The most commonly identified neoplasms are astrocytomas, ependymomas and craniopharyngiomas. Hamartomas of the tuber cinereum account for one in six cases of isosexual precocious puberty in girls and half of the cases in boys. These congenital malformations contain fiber bundles, glial cells and gonadotropin-releasing hormone (GnRH)-secreting neurons.

Girls with severe primary hypothyroidism can develop true precocious puberty along with hyperprolactinemia and galactorrhea. These girls have elevated circulating gonadotropins in addition to very high thyroid-stimulating hormone (TSH) levels. The precocious puberty may be the result of direct gonadotropin stimulation of the ovary or activation of the follicle-stimulating hormone (FSH) receptor by the pathologically high TSH. Hyperprolactinemia results from stimulation of pituitary lactotrophs by the excess thyrotropin-releasing hormone (TRH), a potent stimulator of prolactin secretion (Chapter 1).

Occasionally, correction of a long-standing virilizing condition in girls, such as congenital adrenal hyperplasia, will be followed by development of true sexual precocity. This occurs because removal of the excess androgen releases the hypothalamus from negative feedback, thereby permitting GnRH secretion and gonadotropin stimulation of the ovary.

Treatment of true precocious puberty involves recognition and correction of underlying CNS lesions where appropriate and suppression of the pituitary–gonadal axis with a GnRH agonist. GnRH agonists are long-acting analogs of GnRH that occupy its receptors for extended periods of time. Prolonged receptor occupation removes the GnRH pulsatility necessary for gonadotropin release from the pituitary.

Incomplete isosexual precocity

Incomplete isosexual precocity is caused by ovarian or adrenal secretion of estrogen in girls and testicular or adrenal secretion of androgen in boys.

In girls, functionally autonomous ovarian cysts are the most common cause of GnRH-independent precocious puberty. Small (< 1 cm) follicles occur frequently in the prepubertal ovary but rarely secrete significant amounts of estrogen. However, autonomous secretion of

Differential diagnosis of isosexual precocious puberty.

	Serum gonadotropin concentration	LH response to GnRH	Serum sex steroid concentrations	Gonadal size	Miscellaneous
True precocious puberty (premature activation of hypothalamic GnRH pulse generator)	Prominent LH pulses	Pubertal LH response	Pubertal	Normal pubertal	MRI scan to rule out CNS abnomality, bone scan to exclude McCune–Albright syndrome
Incomplete sexual precocity (GnRH independent)					
Girls					
Follicular cysts	Low	Suppressed	Varies	Ovarian enlargement	Exclude McCune–Albright syndrome
Granulosa cell tumor	Low	Suppressed	Very high estradiol	Ovarian enlargement	Tumor may be palpable
Feminizing adrenal tumor	Low	Suppressed	High estradiol and DHEA-S	Prepubertal ovaries	Unilateral adrenal mass
Boys					
Congenital adrenal hyperplasia	Low	Suppressed	High 17-hydroxyprogesterone	Prepubertal testes	
Virilizing adrenal tumors	Low	Suppressed	High DHEA-S	Prepubertal	Unilateral adrenal mass
Leydig/Sertoli cell tumor	Low	Suppressed	High testosterone	Testicular mass	

CNS, central nervous system; DHEA-S, dehydroepiandrosterone sulfate; GnRH, gonadotropin-releasing hormone; LH, luteinizing hormone; MRI, magnetic resonance imaging.

estradiol by the granulosa cells contained in the cyst wall can occur in larger cysts, and serum estradiol concentrations appear to correlate directly with cyst size. Progestin therapy can reduce the size of the cysts and prevent their recurrence.

In contrast to ovarian cysts which are a common cause of precocious puberty, solid stromal cell tumors of the ovary are a rare cause. Juvenile granulosa or theca cell tumors secrete very large amount of estrogen compared to the functional cysts.

Two inherited syndromes, Peutz–Jeghers and McCune–Albright, are associated with isosexual precocious puberty. Peutz–Jeghers syndrome, which is defined by the appearance of mucocutaneous pigmentation and gastrointestinal polyposis, may also include gonadal sex cord tumors. McCune–Albright syndrome includes hyperpigmented café-au-lait spots, progressive polyostotic fibrous dysplasia of the bones and GnRH-independent sexual precocity. Hyperplasia or adenomas of multiple endocrine glands may occur. The disorder is caused by activating mutations in a guanosine triphosphate-activated $G_s\alpha$ signal transduction protein linked to many of the peptide hormone receptors. These mutations occur in postzygotic somatic cells, thereby accounting for the patchy and unpredictable tissue distribution of abnormalities. Sexual precocity in girls with McCune–Albright syndrome occurs because of estrogen secretion from luteinized follicular cysts. Patients with McCune–Albright syndrome can progress normally through GnRH-dependent puberty because of the lack of CNS involvement.

In boys, incomplete precocious puberty is rare. It can be caused by mild forms of congenital adrenal hyperplasia or other causes of excess adrenal androgen production such as adenomas or cancers. Most virilizing adrenal tumors in children secrete excess amounts of dehydroepiandrosterone sulfate (DHEA-S), which are converted to more potent androgens (Chapter 3). Leydig cell tumors of the testes that produce testosterone are also rare.

Iatrogenic sexual precocity

Breast development has been reported in girls and boys after exposure to estrogens found in tonics, lotions, creams and estrogen-contaminated meat.

Virilizing precocious puberty in girls

Most girls with contrasexual precocious puberty will develop pubic hair or hirsutism. The most common cause is a mild form of 21-hydroxylase deficiency which is present in 0.1–1.0% of the population. This condition is associated with later virilization than classic congenital adrenal hyperplasia and may also present as premature adrenarche, polycystic ovarian disease or postpubertal oligoamenorrhea. The presence of baseline mild elevations in the precursor molecule, 17-hydroxyprogesterone, accompanied by an exaggerated release of 17-hydroxyprogesterone to adrenocorticotropic hormone (ACTH) stimulation will make the diagnosis. Rarely, 11β-hydroxylase deficiency or 3β-hydroxysteroid dehydrogenase deficiency will cause virilizing precocious puberty in girls.

Virilizing adrenal tumors that occur in young girls are very aggressive and usually fatal if malignant. Ovarian Leydig or Sertoli cell tumors, the most common virilizing neoplasm in women, are rare causes of virilizing precocious puberty.

Feminizing precocious puberty in boys

Contrasexual precosity is much less common in boys than in girls. Boys with feminizing precocious puberty will exhibit gynecomastia as well as accelerated linear growth. The presence of prepubertal size testes strongly suggests an adrenal or testicular source for the estrogen. A rare cause of prepubertal feminization is extraglandular aromatization of androstenedione. Gynecomastia has occasionally been seen with congenital adrenal hyperplasia in boys. Feminizing testicular tumors have been reported in boys with Peutz–Jeghers syndrome.

27 Delayed or absent puberty

Classification of delayed or absent puberty.

Constitutional delay in growth and puberty

Hypogonadotropic hypogonadism
CNS disorders
    Congenital malformations
    Destructive lesions
       Tumors
       Radiation therapy
Kallman syndrome (isolated gonadotropin deficiency)
Multiple pituitary hormone deficiencies
Miscellaneous disorders
Prader–Willi syndrome
Functional gonadotropin deficiency
    Chronic systemic disease and malnutrition
    Hypothyroidism
    Cushing's disease
    Diabetes mellitus
    Hyperprolactinemia
    Anorexia nervosa
    Psychogenic amenorrhea
    Exercise-induced amenorrhea
    Fertile eunuch syndrome

Hypergonadotropic hypogonadism
Gonadal dysgenesis
    Turner syndrome
    Klinefelter syndrome
    XX and XY gonadal dysgenesis
Other forms of primary gonadal failure
Disorders of gonadal steroidogenesis = congenital adrenal hyperplasia (CAH)
    Lipoid CAH
    17α-Hydroxylase/17,20-lyase deficiency
    3β-Hydroxysteroid dehydrogenase deficiency
    20,22-Desmolase deficiency

Delayed puberty is defined as the absence of secondary sexual characteristics at age 13 in girls and 16 in boys (Chapters 10 and 11). Delayed puberty may result from: (i) a **constitutional delay** accompanying a growth delay without underlying pathology; (ii) disorders of the hypothalamus or pituitary leading to inadequate gonadotropin secretion (**hypogonadotropic hypogonadism**); and (iii) disorders of the gonads preventing adequate sex steroid secretion (**hypergonadotropic hypogonadism**). In girls, secondary sexual characteristics may develop without progression to menarche. Primary amenorrhea in the presence of female secondary sexual characteristics constitutes a special subset of disorders described in Chapter 28.

It is important to diagnose and treat delayed or absent puberty for several reasons: (i) serious underlying conditions may be present; (ii) a child-like phenotype has profound social implications for the teenager and young adult; and (iii) the prolonged absence of gonadal steroids leads to osteopenia, a failure of normal bone formation. Osteopenia is associated with risk of fractures in weight-bearing bones such as vertebrae, hips and long bones. Treatment is directed at correction of underlying disorders and hormone replacement with estrogen and progesterone or testosterone if hypogonadism persists.

Constitutional delay
The diagnosis of constitutional delay is one of exclusion of other causes of delayed puberty. It is marked by a growth velocity and gonadotropin-releasing hormone (GnRH) secretory pattern that is appropriate for the individual's bone age. In girls, it has been observed that puberty begins once a bone age of 12 years has been reached.

Hypogonadotropic hypogonadism
Hypogonadotropic hypogonadism is characterized by **deficient pulsatile GnRH, follicle-stimulating hormone (FSH) or luteinizing hormone (LH) secretion** resulting in sexual infantilism. GnRH deficiencies arise via three general mechanisms: genetic and developmental defects of the hypothalamus and destructive lesions involving the hypothalamus or pituitary stalk.

The best characterized and most common of the genetic defects producing hypogonadotropic hypogonadism is **Kallman syndrome**. Kallman syndrome consists of a GnRH deficiency associated with hyposmia and hypoplasia of the olfactory lobes of the brain. It is inherited either as a X-linked recessive or an autosomal dominant trait with variable penetrance that is much more common in boys than in girls. The associated abnormalities appear to arise because of failure of fetal GnRH neurosecretory neurons to migrate from where they originate in the olfactory placode to the medial basal hypothalamus. Half of Kallman syndrome patients have mutations in the *KAL* gene on chromosome Xp22.3 that encodes an extracellular matrix protein which regulates axonal pathfinding and cellular adhesion.

Other developmental defects that are associated with delayed or absent puberty due to hypogonadotropic hypogonadism are those that involve midline central nervous system defects that also involve the optic tract. Often other hypothalamic–pituitary functions are abnormal in these patients. A familial form of isolated gonadotropin deficiency has also been described. Unlike most other forms of hypogonadotropic hypogonadism in which growth-hormone is also deficient, familial isolated gonadotropin deficiency has normal height for bone age.

Central nervous system tumors result in delayed puberty more often than precocious puberty. Most of these neoplasms are extrasellar and interfere with production of or delivery of the pituitary trophic hormones to the pituitary gland. Deficiencies in multiple pituitary hormones are common. Of the tumors, craniopharyngioma is the most common cause of delayed or absent puberty. Craniopharyngiomas develop from cells within Rathke's pouch, which is the developmental anlagen of the anterior pituitary. They are almost always located in or near the hypothalamus or pituitary. Other pituitary tumors, such as prolactin-secreting adenomas, which are common in adults, are rare in prepubertal children. They are seen, however, in teenagers and are a cause of primary amenorrhea in the presence of secondary sexual characteristics in girls. Germ-cell tumors and neurofibromas of the CNS that develop as part of von Recklinghausen syndrome are both associated with sexual infantilism.

Functional gonadotropin deficiencies can arise from a large array of chronic diseases, from malnutrition and from psychiatric disorders. Girls seem more sensitive than boys to the effects of malnutrition. In girls, a reduction in body weight to less than 80% of ideal can be associated with delayed or arrested puberty. By contrast, starvation of famine proportions is necessary to interfere with male puberty.

Anorexia nervosa is a serious psychiatric disorder characterized by a distorted body image and obsessive fear of obesity associated with food avoidance. It can cause severe, and sometimes fatal, weight loss. While not restricted by age or gender, anorexia nervosa is far more common in girls than in boys and most often begins during adolescence. Anorexia nervosa is associated with delayed puberty, primary amenorrhea or secondary amenorrhea depending on the girl's age at onset. The hypogonadotropic hypogonadism of anorexia nervosa is related in part to the weight loss associated with the disorder, but in postpubertal girls, secondary amenorrhea may precede severe weight loss. Affected individuals will have a reversion of LH secretion to a prepubertal circadian rhythm. Recovery of normal weight will correct many of the coexisting endocrine and metabolic abnormalities (low cortisol and triiodothyronine, increased growth hormone and decreased IGF-I and blunted pituitary response to trophic hormones) while the amenorrhea may last much longer. A primary hypothalamic origin of the amenorrhea is suggested from the finding that bulimia nervosa, a variant of anorexia nervosa associated with food gorging, induced vomiting and laxative abuse, produces amenorrhea unassociated with weight loss.

Intense exercise and athletic training may delay or arrest puberty due to inhibition of GnRH secretion. Again, this is more common in girls, and distance runners, gymnasts and dancers are at highest risk. Interruption of the intense training by injury advances puberty before weight gain occurs, suggesting a direct effect of the physical activity on GnRH secretion. Female athletes with normal weight gain but less body fat than non-athletic girls (swimmers and ice skaters, for example) are also at risk for hypogonadotropic hypogonadism at puberty.

Hypergonadotropic hypogonadism

Gonadal dysgenesis is the most common cause of hypergonadotropic hypogonadism. Primary gonadal failure results in decreased or absent gonadal steroid secretion. The lack of adequate estrogen or androgen, in turn, causes elevated FSH and LH secretion secondary to the lack of negative feedback.

Klinefelter syndrome is the most common cause of gonadal dysgenesis, occuring in 1 in 500–1000 of all phenotypic boys. Typical features of the Klinefelter phenotype are a eunuch-like habitus, gynecomastia and small testes. The testes of most Klinefelter patients have a distinctly limited capacity to secrete testosterone. The Leydig cells do not respond normally to LH or FSH stimulation; plasma testosterone levels range from 10% of normal in severely eunuchoid boys to about 50% of normal in the less severely affected. Estrogen production is also elevated for the amount of testosterone produced, explaining the frequent finding of gynecomastia. Boys with testosterone levels in the low normal range will demonstrate puberty and normal height. Boys with extremely low testosterone will be very tall because of the failure of the epiphyses to close in a timely fashion. Most Klinefelter men have pubic hair because of adrenal androgen stimulation.

Boys with Klinefelter syndrome also show a progressive loss of spermatogenic activity in the testes after puberty. In normal pubertal boys, about 80% of the seminiferous tubules will have spermatogonia. In Klinefelter boys, only about 20% of tubules will have germ cells; this percentage will decline as the tubules progressively sclerose. Adult men with Klinefelter syndrome are infertile and most will need androgen replacement therapy to obtain or maintain an adult male phenotype.

Ninety per cent of men with Klinefelter syndrome have a **47,XXY karyotype**. Other patterns, including an array of extra X states, mosaicisms and 46,XX with translocation of the male sex-determining region (SRY) onto the X chromosome (Chapter 5.1), account for the other 10%. The mosaics account for the largest proportion of men with some testicular function. Fertile 46,XY mosaics have been reported.

Turner syndrome is the second most common form of gonadal dysgenesis, occuring in about 1 in every 5000 liveborn girls. Typical features of the Turner phenotype include short stature, short webbed neck, micrognathia, broad shield-like chest, anomalies of the left side of the heart (coarctation of the aorta, aortic stenosis, bicuspid aortic valve and dissecting aortic aneurysms) and renal and gastrointestinal anomalies. The uterus and Fallopian tubes are present but remain infantile due to lack of estrogen stimulation from the connective tissue streaks that replace the ovaries (streak gonads). External genitalia and gender orientation are female.

Turner syndrome typically is associated with a **45,X karyotype** although mosaicism and structural abnormalities of the X chromosome are also common. Mosaicism and structural abnormalities account for the varied phenotypes reported with the syndrome. The phenotypes seen with Turner syndrome range from that described above to both normal males and females. The systemic nature of the abnormalities seen with complete absence of the second sex chromosome is attested to by the observation that 99% of conceptuses with the 45,X karyotype spontaneously abort (miscarry).

Patients with Turner syndrome are usually smaller at birth, grow normally for the first few years after infancy and then grow slowly again, failing to demonstrate a pubertal growth spurt. The defect in growth appears to be related to the single copy of a gene on the X chromosome known as *PHOG* or *SHOX*. *PHOG* is a transcription factor expressed in osteoblasts.

Mosaicism involving the Y chromosome may result in phenotypes with ambiguous genitalia or normal male external genitalia in addition to the classic Turner phenotype described above. Gonadal structures range from a streak gonad to functioning testes. Individuals with a Y cell line or abnormalities involving the Y chromosome are at risk for neoplastic transformation. The gonads should be removed at the time of diagnosis for this reason.

The final large category of disorders causing hypergonadotropic hypogonadism includes the **genetic disorders of steroidogenesis**. Because most of these autosomal recessive disorders also affect adrenal steroid biosynthesis, they are more commonly known as the **congenital adrenal hyperplasia (CAH) syndromes**. The CAH syndromes associated with delayed puberty are listed in the table on the facing page. All these enzyme defects occur in the steroidogenic pathway between cholesterol and testosterone. They are rare causes of delayed puberty.

28 Amenorrhea

Causes of amenorrhea.

Hypothalamic disturbances
Primary hypothalamic lesions
   Kallman syndrome
Secondary hypothalamic lesions
   CNS tumors
Abnormal CNS–hypothalamic interaction
   Anorexia nervosa
   Exercise-induced amenorrhea

Primary pituitary disturbances
Sheehan syndrome (pituitary apoplexy)
Pituitary adenomas
Pituitary tumors
Empty sella syndrome

Secondary pituitary disturbances
Inappropriate gonadal steroid feedback
   Pregnancy
   Contraceptive steroids
   Constant estrogen exposure
   Estrogen excess
      Estrogen-producing tumors
      Aromatase excess
   Estrogen deficiency
      Gene mutations in estrogen receptor
      Aromatase deficiency
   Androgen excess
      Androgen-producing tumors
      Functional excess (adrenal or ovarian)
Inappropriate feedback from other sources
   Polycystic ovary syndrome (PCOS)
   Cushing syndrome
   Hypo- and hyperthyroidism
   Lactation
   Hyperprolactinemia
   Growth hormone excess
   Malnutrition

Gonadal abnormalities
Gonadal failure
   Gonadal dysgenesis
   Menopause
   Ovarian ablation or removal
Gene mutation in LH and FSH receptors

End-organ abnormalities
Uterus
   Müllerian agenesis
   Surgical removal of the uterus
   Endometrial ablation
   Asherman syndrome
Vagina
   Imperforate hymen
   Vaginal septum
Other
   Complete androgen insensitivity (testicular feminization)

CNS, central nervous system; FSH, follicle-stimulating hormone; LH, luteinizing hormone.

Overview

Amenorrhea is defined as failure to menstruate by age 16 (**primary amenorrhea**) or the absence of menstrual bleeding for at least 3 months in a woman who has previously had periodic menstruation regardless of prior frequency or regularity (**secondary amenorrhea**). The distinction has traditionally been emphasized because of the higher incidence of genetic and anatomic abnormalities among young women with primary amenorrhea. It is still useful conceptually to distinguish between primary and secondary amenorrhea because of several unique disorders that will be found only in patients with one or the other; however, it should be recognized that there is much more overlap in the origins and pathophysiology of the two entities than was originally appreciated. For example, Turner syndrome is a common genetic cause of primary amenorrhea, yet some patients with Turner syndrome have sufficient ovarian reserve to undergo secondary sexual development and menarche before complete ovarian failure results in secondary amenorrhea. Other young women with chronic anovulation due to functional disorders will be classified with primary amenorrhea if the onset of the disorder is at puberty. It is more useful to assess the degree to which secondary sexual characteristics have developed in girls with absent menses. Failure of breast and pubic hair development is a sign of delayed or absent puberty in girls and represents a specific subset of reproductive abnormalities (Chapter 27).

As can be seen in the table, the causes of amenorrhea are extensive and involve all levels of the hypothalamic–pituitary–gonadal–end-organ axis. In order to avoid confusion, it is useful to note that amenorrhea can be divided broadly into two broad categories of abnormalities. The first and largest category, by far, involves chronic anovulation: the failure to generate cyclic estrogen and progesterone leads to absent or highly irregular sloughing of an inappropriately stimulated endometrium (Chapters 9 and 13). Chronic anovulation results from four general pathophysiologic mechanisms: (i) failure of the hypothalamus to generate a cyclic gonadotropin-releasing hormone (GnRH) signal to the pituitary gland; (ii) failure of the pituitary to respond to an appropriate signal; (iii) failure of the normal sex steroid feedback mechanisms to permit a midcycle LH surge; and (iv) interference with gonadal steroid feedback by other endocrine systems. The second, much smaller, category includes end-organ abnormalities that interfere with the ability of these organs to respond to normal cyclic ovarian steroid production and produce visible endometrial bleeding.

Diagnosis of the underlying cause of amenorrhea involves sequential determination of the function of each compartment (uterus and vagina, ovaries, pituitary and hypothalamus). Treatment is directed toward correction of the underlying problem whenever possible so that menses resume. If it is not possible to establish or restore menstruation, it is very important to assess the hormonal status of the untreated individuals. Women who are hypoestrogenic are at increased risk for osteoporosis (Chapter 21) and women who have chronic unopposed estrogen stimulation of their endometrium are at risk for endometrial cancer (Chapter 40). Hormonal therapy to avoid these consequences must be considered in all amenorrheic women.

1 PRIMARY AMENORRHEA

The etiologies of primary amenorrhea are best understood if categorized by: (i) the presence or absence of breast development; (ii) the presence or absence of the cervix and uterus; and (iii) circulating follicle-stimulating hormone (FSH) levels. An algorithm for evaluating the girl or woman with primary amenorrhea is presented in the figure below. Not surprisingly, abnormalities in each of the four compartments are associated with primary amenorrhea.

In order of descending frequency, the most common causes of primary amenorrhea are gonadal dysgenesis, physiologic delay of puberty, Müllerian agenesis, transverse vaginal septum or imperforate hymen, Kallman syndrome, anorexia nervosa and hypopituitarism. Complete androgen insensitivity, while much rarer than Müllerian agenesis, must be considered in any young woman who has breasts but no uterus. All girls or women with primary amenorrhea and an elevated FSH must have a karyotype performed to determine if a Y chromosome or even a piece of a Y chromosome is present. The presence of any Y chromosome genes in an intra-abdominal gonad, regardless of its phenotype, confers a risk that a germ-cell tumor will develop in the gonad and it must be removed.

Gonadal dysgenesis with a pure 45,X karyotype can usually be diagnosed because of the other physical features of Turner syndrome (Chapter 27). Other abnormalities of the sex chromosomes such as 45,X/46,XX and other mosaics as well as 46,XY with a missing SRY locus (Chapter 5.1) can also cause amenorrhea. **Müllerian agenesis**, known also as the Mayer–Rokitansky–Kuster–Hauser syndrome, involves complete absence of the female internal genitalia including the vagina, uterus and Fallopian tubes in a chromosomally normal female. Its biologic cause is unknown. **Transverse vaginal septa** are thought to result from failure of the vaginal plate to resorb at the site where the Müllerian ducts fuse with it to form the cervix (Chapter 25). **Kallman syndrome** is a developmental abnormality of the central nervous system in which the neurosecretory cells destined to become the GnRH pulse generator fail to migrate from their origins in the olfactory placode to the median basal hypothalamus (Chapter 27). Individuals with Kallman syndrome also cannot smell because of the absence of the olfactory neurons that develop from the same anlagen. **Anorexia nervosa** and the consequent hypothalamic suppression can cause delayed or absent puberty if the disorder begins in childhood, primary amenorrhea if it begins during puberty, or secondary amenorrhea if it begins later in adolescence. **Hypopituitarism** most commonly results from central nervous system tumors and can present as either absent or delayed puberty or amenorrhea alone depending on the rate of tumor growth. **Complete androgen insensitivity, or testicular feminization** as it used to be called, is a rare X-linked disorder caused by mutations in the androgen receptor that make it unresponsive to androgen. As a result of the lack of androgen activity at both central and peripheral target tissues, there is failure of the genitalia to masculinize during embryogenesis followed by failure of androgen feedback on FSH production. These phenotypic girls develop breasts at puberty because of the adequate estrogen production by the overstimulated testes but cannot menstruate because of the lack of a uterus.

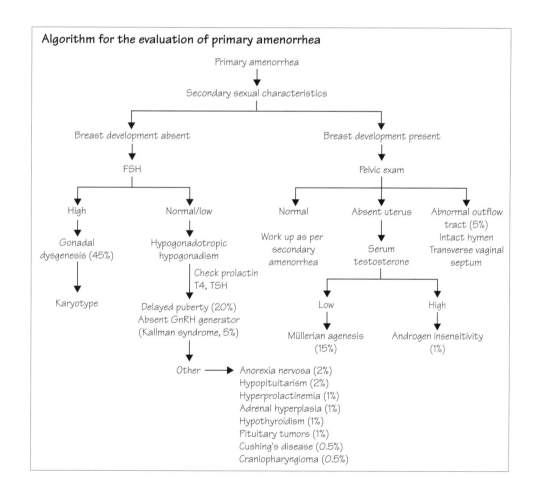

2 SECONDARY AMENORRHEA

Most secondary amenorrhea results from anovulation. The most common reason for secondary amenorrhea is **pregnancy**; this etiology should be evaluated before considering any other possible causes. After pregnancy, the most common causes of secondary amenorrhea are: (i) polycystic ovary syndrome; (ii) functional hypothalamic disorders such as anorexia nervosa, stress and exercise; (iii) hyperprolactinemia; (iv) premature ovarian failure; (v) Asherman syndrome; (vi) thyroid dysfunction; (vii) congenital adrenal hyperplasia, Cushing syndrome and obesity; (viii) empty sella syndrome; and (ix) Sheehan syndrome. An algorithm for evaluating the woman with secondary amenorrhea is presented in the figure below.

The polycystic ovary syndrome (PCOS) is the single most common cause of chronic anovulatory amenorrhea. It is a clinical disorder characterized by hirsutism, acne, amenorrhea or oligoamenorrhea and enlarged polycystic ovaries. The pathophysiology of PCOS involves: (i) elevated circulating luteinizing hormone (LH) and an increased LH/FSH ratio due to an exaggeration of pulsatile GnRH secretion; and (ii) insulin resistance secondary to defects in insulin signaling for intracellular glucose transport and lipolysis. The mechanism for the exaggerated GnRH pulse frequency and amplitude is not yet known, but its appearance at puberty in these women suggests that it is an intrinsic, primary pathogenic defect. The result of the exaggerated GnRH pulsatility is an increase in LH secretion and a relative deficiency in FSH. The theca cells in the ovary respond to the LH by increasing cholesterol conversion to androgens (Chapter 3). The relative deficiency in FSH then fails to adequately stimulate production of the enzyme aromatase and conversion of androgen to estrogen is poor, leading to hyperandrogenism. In turn, the hyperandrogenism causes local follicular arrest and anovulation in the ovary and hirsuitism through excess stimulation of sensitive hair follicles (Chapter 29). Microscopically, the ovaries in PCOS are enlarged because of hyperplasia of the theca-stromal cells surrounding an increased number of primary and secondary follicles.

Insulin deficiency is as important to the syndrome of PCOS as is the abnormality in the GnRH pulse generator. The cellular defect in glucose transport results in transient hyperglycemia and reactive hyperinsulinemia. Insulin synergizes with LH in stimulating theca cell androgen production while inhibiting hepatic production of sex hormone-binding globulin (SHBG) at the same time. The net result is an increase in circulating androgen free to act on its target cells. The cellular lipolytic defect in PCOS appears to be due to a reduced β-adrenoceptor density on adipocytes which leads to increased fat storage and predisposes the woman to obesity. Obesity, which is present in half of women with PCOS, further amplifies the abnormalities of insulin resistance and hyperinsulinemia. A role for leptin in the obese PCOS patient is hypothesized, but is not clear at this time. Obese women with PCOS are at significant risk for developing type II diabetes and cardiovascular disease as a result of the amplified insulin resistance.

In addition to the direct actions of insulin upon the theca cells and liver to produce excess androgen activity, other parts of the somatotropic or growth axis appear involved in PCOS as well. The

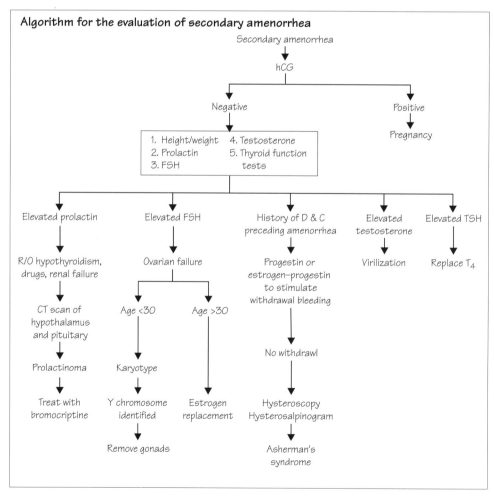

Algorithm for the evaluation of secondary amenorrhea

somatotropic axis is driven primarily by growth hormone (GH) and nutritional status. The insulin-like growth factors (IGFs), their binding proteins (IGFBPs) and the IGF-1 and IGF-2 receptors are the peripheral mediators of GH. Both GH and the IGFs act within the ovary to enhance steroidogenesis by the theca and granulosa cells. Non-obese PCOS patients demonstrate an exaggeration in GH pulse amplitude that is similar to the exaggerated GnRH pulses seen in the disorder. Obese patients with PCOS show a blunting of GH secretion. Insulin, which interacts with the IGF system at multiple levels, notably in binding to the IGF-1 receptor, will mimic the GH excess. In both cases, increased somatotropic activity in the ovary appears to enhance androgen production.

At least 50% of women with PCOS also show functional adrenal hyperandrogenism. Indeed PCOS has many features in common with late-onset congenital adrenal hyperplasia (CAH) including amenorrhea and hirsuitism. The exact nature of the adrenal dysfunction in PCOS is not yet elucidated, but evidence points to an increase in P450c17 activities in the zona reticularis of the adrenal cortex. This is the same enzyme that is stimulated by LH, insulin and IGF-1 in the ovary to produce androgens. PCOS patients with functional adrenal hyperandrogenism demonstrate a prompt and excessive responsiveness of adrenal androgen production to adrenocorticotropic hormone (ACTH) stimulation in much the same way that LH responsiveness is exaggerated. This has lead to the hypothesis that, in these patients, an exaggerated adrenarche at puberty triggers the onset of PCOS by the following mechanism: exaggerated adrenarche produces increased serum androstenedione which is converted extragonadally to the weak estrogen estrone. The estrone, in turn, exerts a premature and pathologic trophic effect on the reproductive axis, leading to PCOS at puberty.

Treatment of PCOS is directed toward reducing insulin resistance, establishing ovulation when fertility is desired and preventing the development of endometrial hyperplasia and cancer from the unopposed estrogen activity during prolonged periods of anovulation. Antiandrogens can be also be used to mitigate the androgenic effects such as hirsutism.

Functional hypothalamic disorders include all those disorders associated with decreased GnRH pulse frequency and amplitude. The higher CNS input to the pulse generator can be disrupted by the psychogenic starvation of anorexia nervosa, strenuous exercise and stress. Infiltrative diseases of the hypothalamus like lymphoma and histiocytosis, while rare, also cause disruption of GnRH secretion.

Amenorrhea resulting from **excessive prolactin secretion** can arise from a variety of abnormalities including prolactin secreting micro- and macroadenomas, hypothyroidism and a variety of medications. Hyperprolactinemia is covered in detail in Chapter 30.

Premature ovarian failure is the cessation of menses before the age of 40 in the absence of any demonstrable genetic abnormality. It accounts for about 10% of the cases of secondary amenorrhea. Women with premature ovarian failure typically have the symptom complex of amenorrhea, elevated gonadotropin levels and decreased circulating estrogen. Many will also have hot flashes. The exact cause of the disorder has not been elucidated. In a number of cases, associated autoimmune disease such as Hashimoto thyroiditis, Addison's disease, hypoparathyroidism or myasthenia gravis is present. Premature ovarian failure may be part of a polyendocrine syndrome. While antibodies to both gonadotropins and gonadotropin receptors have been found in many of these patients, some also appear to have genetic mutations in the LH and FSH receptors. In some of these women, ovarian failure is not permanent and pregnancies have ensued.

Asherman syndrome is the name given to a condition in which intrauterine synechiae or adhesions occlude the uterine cavity. Typically, the condition develops after a postpartum curettage of the uterus is performed for heavy bleeding or infection. It is believed that the removal of an additional layer of endometrium destroys the basal crypts and glands from which the endometrium regenerates postpartum. Scarring across the denuded endometrium can completely obliterate the uterine cavity. Milder degrees of scarring can also be associated with amenorrhea, suggesting some local paracrine dysfunction as well.

Hypothyroidism is associated with menstrual irregularities and amenorrhea. Two mechanisms are potentially involved. The first is a direct effect of thyroid hormone deficiency upon ovarian steroidogenesis. Thyroxine has been shown to increase the secretion of both estrogen and progesterone from granulosa cells in culture. In addition, primary hypothyroidism is associated with increased hypothalamic secretion of thyrotropin-releasing hormone (TRH). TRF stimulates prolactin secretion; the hyperprolactinemia in turn interferes with pulsatile GnRH secretion (Chapter 30).

Congenital adrenal hyperplasia, Cushing syndrome and obesity all are associated with excess androgen production. Although the androgens produced by the adrenal gland (DHEA and DHEA-S; Chapter 3) are relatively weak androgens, their presence in pathologic amounts can lead to significant androgenic effects in the body. This occurs largely because of their conversion to more potent androgens and estrogens in peripheral tissues such as the adipocyte. Such non-cyclic, gonadotropin-independent sex steroid secretion in women will interfere with normal cyclic secretion of FSH and LH by the pituitary.

Empty sella syndrome refers to an idiopathic condition of the sella turcica in which the pituitary gland is flattened and the sella appears enlarged and empty. Some patients with an apparently empty sella will have headaches and no endocrine dysfunction while others will have single or multiple endocrinopathies including gonadotropin deficiencies and hyperprolactinemia. The cause is unknown.

Sheehan syndrome is the name given to a specific condition leading to pituitary apoplexy and stroke. Sheehan described a condition of panhypopituitarism resulting from postpartum hemorrhage and shock. While it is rare to see the complete syndrome in modern obstetric practice, a discrete form in which only parts of the pituitary are affected is still occasionally seen. These patients have demonstrated that the impairment in pituitary function following postpartum pituitary infarction appears to be, in decreasing order of frequency: GH, LH/FSH, ACTH, prolactin and TSH secreting ability.

29 Hirsutism and androgenetic alopecia

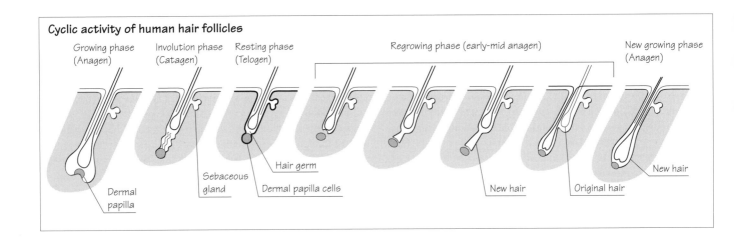

Cyclic activity of human hair follicles

Growing phase (Anagen) — Involution phase (Catagen) — Resting phase (Telogen) — Regrowing phase (early-mid anagen) — New growing phase (Anagen)

Dermal papilla — Sebaceous gland — Hair germ — Dermal papilla cells — New hair — Original hair — New hair

Hirsutism and androgenetic alopecia (commonly known as male-pattern baldness) result from androgen activity on hair follicles that are not normally responsive to androgens. While both demonstrate wide ethnic and cultural variations in acceptance, both conditions are of considerable cosmetic concern to some individuals. In addition, hirsutism in women may be a sign of a serious underlying disorder such as chronic anovulation or an androgen-producing tumor.

Biology of the human hair follicle

Hair is an appendage of skin. The functional unit of hair, the pilosebaceous unit, is composed of the individual hair follicle plus its attached sebaceous gland. Both skin and the pilosebaceous unit are sensitive to hormones, especially androgens.

Human hair follicles are divided into three types depending on the size and depth of the follicle and the characteristics of the hair they produce. Vellus hair follicles are small and shallow in depth. They produce fine and minimally pigmented hairs. Vellus hair follicles are found all over the body, with the exception of the scalp, eyebrows and eyelashes. Medium hair follicles are larger in caliber than vellus follicles and extend deeper into the dermis. These follicles produce slightly heavier pigmented hairs. Medium hair follicles are found on the upper arms and lower legs and in the transition zones between vellus and thick (terminal) hair such as the scalp hairline. Terminal hair follicles are the largest hair follicles. They produce thick pigmented hair. Terminal follicles extend through the dermis into the cutaneous adipose layer. Normally, terminal hair follicles are found in the scalp, axillae and pubic area of both men and women and on the face and chest of men. Vellus hair follicles in certain anatomic locations, notably the face, breasts, lower abdomen and anterior thighs of women, can be converted into terminal follicles under the influence of excess androgen.

All three types of hair follicles undergo cyclic patterns of growth and regression called anagen, catagen and telogen (see figure above). The lengths of these cycles are intrinsic to each hair follicle type and the body region in which it is located. For example, anagen lasts 3 years for terminal hair follicles on the scalp but only 3 months on the upper lip. In addition to the length of anagen, growth is related to the percentage of

hair in anagen in a region at any one time and to the actual rate of linear growth of the hair itself. Hormonal control of hair growth is exclusively through acceleration of the rate of entry of hair follicles into anagen from telogen.

The pilosebaceous units of the terminal hair follicles regulate androgen stimulation of hair growth. The sebaceous glands contain the enzyme 5α-reductase, which converts other androgen precursors to the potent androgen dihydrotestosterone (DHT). DHT produced locally within the pilosebaceous gland stimulates terminal hair growth through its action on the matrix cells surrounding the dermal papillae (see figure below).

During puberty, adrenal and testicular androgens convert vellus and medium hair follicles into terminal hair follicles in specific areas of the body. Pubic and axillary hair follicles are quite sensitive to androgens and form terminal hair in response to the weak adrenal androgens

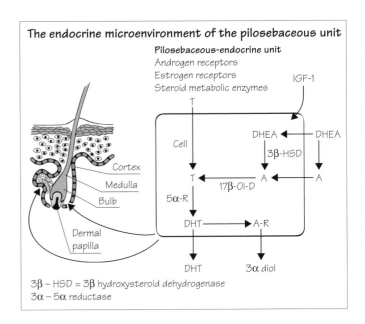

The endocrine microenvironment of the pilosebaceous unit

Pilosebaceous-endocrine unit
Androgen receptors
Estrogen receptors
Steroid metabolic enzymes

IGF-1

Cortex — Medulla — Bulb — Dermal papilla

Cell — T — DHEA ← DHEA — 3β-HSD — T ← A ← A — 17β-Ol-D — 5α-R — DHT → A-R — DHT — 3α diol

3β – HSD = 3β hydroxysteroid dehydrogenase
3α – 5α reductase

secreted at adrenarche (adrenal puberty; Chapter 10). Facial and body hair is relatively insensitive to androgen and normally responds only to the high levels of testicular androgens secreted after puberty in men.

Hirsutism

Hirsutism in women is a common clinical condition manifested by excessive hair growth in a male pattern. It results from increased androgen stimulation of specific vellus hair follicles, which then become terminal hair follicles with dense pigmented hair growth on the face, back and chest.

The androgen increase can occur because of excessive androgen production by the ovaries, adrenals or other extraglandular sources such as tumors, or by local biotransformation within the hair follicle. Two conditions, the polycystic ovary syndrome (PCOS) and 'idiopathic' hirsutism, are responsible for 95% of the cases of hirsutism. Hirsute women with PCOS are usually anovulatory as well.

Because most vellus hair follicles are relatively insensitive to androgens, prolonged stimulation by high levels of androgen is necessary for hirsutism to develop. Thus, hirsutism resulting from PCOS will be very slow to develop and appears after menstrual irregularities are present. The rapid development of hirsutism is indicative of very high androgen exposure and is more typical of androgen-secreting tumors.

Idiopathic hirsutism develops in women with normal circulating levels of ovarian and adrenal androgens. It results from excessive 5α-reductase activity in the pilosebaceous unit. Idiopathic hirsutism is often familial. Differences in 5α-reductase activity may explain much of the racial and ethnic differences in hair density and distribution in men and women.

Management of the hirsute woman is directed toward identifying the underlying etiology and correcting it whenever possible. Effective treatments involve either generalized ovarian suppression, which decreases ovarian androgen production, or specific antiandrogen therapy. In women with PCOS who do not desire fertility, long-term use of **combination oral contraceptive pills** will treat both their PCOS and hirsutism. The oral contraceptives appear to act through four separate mechanisms in these patients: (i) suppression of gonadotropin secretion by the pituitary; (ii) reduction of ovarian androgen secretion; (iii) increasing hepatic synthesis of sex hormone-binding globulin (SHBG), thereby decreasing the amount of circulating free androgen; and (iv) inhibition of DHT binding to pilosebaceous androgen receptors. **GnRH agonists** such as leuprolide will also suppress ovarian function and androgen production but require concomitant use of estrogen and progesterone to counter the effects of hypoestrogenism.

Antiandrogen therapy can be either general or specific. **Spironolactone**, an aldosterone antagonist with remarkable structural homology to testosterone, can return ovarian cyclicity and treat hirsutism in PCOS patients. Spironolactone works by two mechanisms in these patients: (i) inhibition of the enzyme complex P450c17 which is required to convert cholesterol to sex steroid precursors in the adrenal and ovary (Chapter 3); and (ii) occupation of the androgen receptors in the hair follicle, thereby preventing DHT binding and action.

Cyproterone acetate is an antiandrogen that has antigonadotropin actions as well. In combination with dexamethasone, it will also restore cyclicity to PCOS women while treating their hirsutism. Cyproterone acetate works by (i) decreasing ovarian androgen production by decreasing gonadotropin release; (ii) reducing 5α-reductase activity in the skin; and (iii) competitively inhibiting DHT binding to its receptors in the hair follicle. Cyproterone acetate is available in Europe and Canada, but not in the United States.

Flutamide is a potent non-steroidal selective antiandrogen that has no progestational, estrogenic, glucocorticoid or antigonadotropic activity. It is very effective in the treatment of hirsutism. **Finasteride**, a selective competitive inhibitor of 5α-reductase, is also effective in treating hirsutism.

Androgenetic alopecia

While typically thought to be a problem for men, androgenetic alopecia actually manifests itself in both sexes. In men, hairline regression begins at the temples followed by progressive hair loss over the top of the head such that only a crown of hair around the ears and occiput remain. In women, androgen-dependent hair loss is usually an extensive overall thinning of the hair over the top of the head and depletion at the crown. Women rarely go completely bald as happens to some men.

Hair loss is a normal part of the aging process and men and women tend to lose it in patterns similar to that seen with androgenetic alopecia. The definition of androgenetic alopecia is patterned hair loss that occurs before the age of 30 years in a man and excessive hair loss on the crown of a woman at any age. There is typically a family history of early balding but the inheritance pattern of the disorder is unclear as is the exact underlying pathophysiology. The absence of the disorder among individuals castrated before puberty and those with androgen insensitivity or 5α-reductase deficiency indicates that DHT activity at the androgen receptor is necessary for the development of androgenetic alopecia.

The best explanation to date for androgenetic alopecia is that DHT in susceptible individuals leads to regression of terminal hair follicles back to vellus follicles in specific areas of the scalp. While men with androgenetic alopecia do not have excessive circulating androgen, the affected hair follicles demonstrate biochemical differences when compared to hairy areas of the scalp. The sebaceous glands in the bald areas have greater 3β-hydroxysteroid dehydrogenase (3β-HSD) activity and greater androgen-binding activity than unaffected areas. 3β-HSD is rate-limiting in the formation of androstenedione and testosterone and partially controls the amount of androgen available for reduction to DHT. The sebaceous glands of affected terminal hairs appear to hypertrophy before hair growth ceases and androgen metabolism to DHT may be enhanced in the enlarged glands. Overstimulation of the hair matrix in the dermal papilla by androgens then leads to death of the hair follicle.

Treatment of androgenetic alopecia aims to stop regression of the terminal hair follicles back to the vellus type. This may be accomplished through the use of selective antiandrogens or chemical agents. Spironolactone and cyproterone acetate are effective but are associated with unacceptable reductions in circulating androgen levels. The 5α-reductase inhibitor, **finasteride**, is the most specific treatment currently available. It reduces the amount of DHT available to stimulate the susceptible terminal hair matrix cells and prevents their untimely regression to vellus hair while leaving other androgen activities intact. **Minoxidil**, a potent vasodilator, can regenerate terminal hair growth in about 40% of men when applied topically to affected areas. The mechanism of action of minoxidil is unknown.

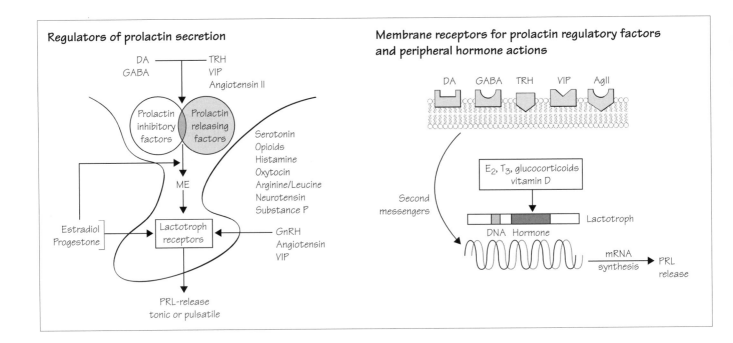

Regulators of prolactin secretion

Membrane receptors for prolactin regulatory factors and peripheral hormone actions

Hyperprolactinemia resulting from inappropriate prolactin secretion is a common clinical problem. It is the third most frequently diagnosed cause of chronic anovulation and secondary amenorrhea. There are many causes for this condition; some result from serious underlying pathology and others from reversible functional disorders.

Prolactin is a unique pituitary hormone in that its secretion is dominated by tonic inhibition. In addition, it is not regulated by classic negative feedback from its target organs (Chapter 1). The major inhibitor of prolactin secretion is dopamine and the two major stimuli are estrogen and thyrotropin-releasing hormone (TRH). There are numerous other regulators that must be considered when elucidating the mechanisms by which hyperprolactinemia develops.

Regulation of prolactin secretion

Embryonic differentiation of the lactotroph is under the control of the pituitary-specific transcriptional factor Pit-1. In addition to the action of Pit-1 on the prolactin promoter, prolactin gene expression is regulated by dopamine, TRH and estradiol. Dopamine released into the portal system binds to a G_1 protein-coupled receptor and inhibits adenylate cyclase and phospholipase C. Both prolactin synthesis and release are reduced by dopamine acting, in this instance, as a neurohormone rather than as a neurotransmitter. TRH acts through a second lactotroph cell membrane to activate phospholipase C. TRH increases prolactin gene transcription and release of prolactin hormone from its storage granules. The effect of TRH is modulated by thyroid hormone such that decreases in T_3 and T_4 enhance prolactin release and increased concentrations of T_3 and T_4 decrease prolactin secretion. Estradiol acts through a third mechanism, binding first to its nuclear receptor and then as a complex with the response element in the gene. Estradiol also interferes with dopaminergic activation of its receptor

and increases the concentration of TRH receptors on lactotrophs, thereby potentiating the stimulatory effect of the sex steroid.

In addition to dopamine, γ-aminobutyric acid (GABA) and glucocorticoids inhibit prolactin secretion. The mechanism by which GABA acts as a prolactin inhibitory factor is unknown. Glucocorticoids act through nuclear receptors similar to the estrogen receptor to inhibit prolactin gene transcription. Vasoactive peptide (VIP), oxytocin, angiotensin II and serotonin all increase prolactin secretion. VIP acts to increase prolactin secretion both by stimulating oxytocin release via the hypothalamus and by interfering with dopamine inhibition of adenylate cyclase. Angiotensin II (AgII) acts on a specific receptor on the lactotroph and acutely causes prolactin release. It is a more potent secretagogue for prolactin than TRH. Serotonin released by the dorsal raphe nucleus stimulates prolactin independent of dopamine.

In the physiologic state, fine tuning of prolactin secretion is determined by the balance between the prolactin inhibitory factors (PIF) and the prolactin-releasing factors (PRF). Any disorder that alters the secretion of these regulatory compounds will result in altered prolactin secretion. Hyperprolactinemia, regardless of its cause, can interfere with hypothalamic–pituitary function. The net result is hypogonadism with or without galactorrhea. The fact that women with prolactin-induced amenorrhea are hypoestrogenic but do not experience hot flashes suggests that prolactin alters central neurotransmission as one mechanism by which it alters hypothalamic–pituitary function. The most likely site of action is through the hypothalamic dopaminergic and opioid systems that regulate GnRH pulsatility.

Physiologic hyperprolactinemia

Most physiologic hyperprolactinemia is transient and of no clinical consequence. High physiologic concentrations of plasma prolactin occur at night and result from both an intrinsic circadian rhythm and sleep-entrained prolactin release. High protein meals midday, but not in the morning, induce prolactin release through an unknown mechanism. Physical and emotional stress, including exercise, hypoglycemia, anesthesia, and orgasm in women only, are associated with elevations in prolactin secretion. Pregnancy is associated with a marked elevation of prolactin secretion that persists into the immediate postpartum period (Chapter 20). Of all the physiologic hyperprolactinemic states, only lactation is associated with amenorrhea.

Pharmacologic hyperprolactinemia

Hyperprolactinemia can result from medications that interfere with dopaminergic inhibition of the lactotroph. Any drug that decreases the synthesis of dopamine, enhances its metabolism, decreases its reuptake or interferes with its binding to its receptor will reduce the action of dopamine leading to increased prolactin secretion. Galactorrhea, often accompanied by amenorrhea or menstrual irregularities, is a potential side-effect of all the medications listed in the table below.

Pathologic hyperprolactinemia

Hypothalamic lesions that cause hyperprolactinemia typically do so by interfering in some way with dopamine delivery to the pituitary gland. Pituitary causes of hyperprolactinemia most often are tumors. By far the most common is the pituitary prolactin-secreting adenoma. Adenomas are classified into microadenomas, which are less than 1 cm in size and macroadenomas, which are greater than 1 cm. These tumors occur in both men and women, although they are more common in women. In women they cause galactorrhea, amenorrhea, headache and visual field defects. In men they cause headache, visual field changes and impotence. Prolactinomas are usually benign. They are often larger at diagnosis in men than in women because of the relatively late onset of symptoms in men. Adenomas that produce adrenocorticotropic hormone (Cushing disease) and growth hormone (acromegaly) may also cause hyperprolactinemia.

Primary hypothyroidism is associated with increased TRH and TSH secretion in response to the lack of negative feedback by the thyroid hormones. Excessive TRH can override the normal dopamine-dominated inhibition of prolactin secretion through the action of TRH on its receptor on the lactotrophs. A significant proportion of patients with chronic renal failure will have hyperprolactinemia apparently on the basis of serum factors which interfere with dopaminergic inhibition of prolactin synthesis and secretion.

Treatment of hyperprolactinemia is directed toward correction of the underlying cause. A notable exception to this rule is the management of the prolactin-secreting pituitary adenoma. Resection of these tumors is associated with a high frequency of recurrence of the hyperprolactinemia. Patients with prolactinomas are usually treated with the dopamine agonist **bromocriptine**. It is important to remember that both men and women with hyperprolactinemia are hypogonadal due to the associated abnormalities in the hypothalamic–pituitary–gonadal axis and are at risk for osteoporosis (Chapter 21). Therefore, they are treated indefinitely or for as long as the hyperprolactinemia persists.

Galactorrhea

Galactorrhea is breast-milk secretion unassociated with nursing. Galactorrhea is usually associated with hyperprolactinemia or with excessive sensitivity of the breast to normal circulating levels of prolactin. If the galactorrhea is associated with amenorrhea, then hyperprolactinemia is likely to be the cause. If the galactorrhea occurs in the presence of normal ovulatory cycles, then excessive sensitivity of the breast to normal circulating levels of prolactin is more likely. The three most common causes of hyperprolactinemia resulting in galactorrhea are (i) a pituitary adenoma, (ii) medications interfering with dopamine action and (iii) hypothyroidism. Galactorrhea can be suppressed by the use of bromocriptine, the dopamine agonist.

Conditions associated with increased prolactin secretion.	Physiologic causes	Pharmacologic causes	Pathologic causes
	Sleep	Estrogen therapy	Hypothalamic lesions
	Feeding	Anesthesia	Craniopharyngioma
	Exercise	Dopamine receptor blockers	Glioma
	Stress	Domperidone	Granulomas
	Coitus	Haloperidol	Histiocytosis
	Menstrual cycle	Metoclopramide	Sarcoid
	Pregnancy	Phenothiazine	Tuberculosis
	Postpartum	Pimozide	Pituitary stalk transection
	Nursing	Sulpride	Head injury or postsurgical
	Fetal/neonatal	Dopamine reuptake blockers	Irradiation damage
		Nomifensine	Pseudocyesis
		CNS dopamine depleting agents	Pituitary tumors
		Methyldopa	Cushing disease
		Monoamine oxidase inhibitors	Acromegaly
		Reserpine	Prolactinoma
		Inhibitors of dopamine turnover	Non-secreting adenomas
		Opiates	Neural reflexes
		Stimulators of serotonergic system	Chest wall injury
		Amphetamines	Herpes zoster neuritis
		Hallucinogens	Upper abdominal surgery
		Histamine H_2 receptor antagonists	Hypothyroidism
		Cimetidine	Renal failure
		Ranitidine	Ectopic production
		Nizatidine	Bronchogenic carcinoma
		Famotidine	Hypernephroma

31 Sexual dysfunction

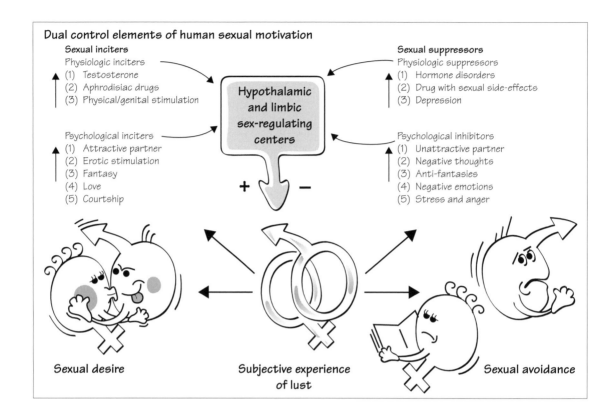

Dual control elements of human sexual motivation

Sexual inciters

Physiologic inciters
(1) Testosterone
(2) Aphrodisiac drugs
(3) Physical/genital stimulation

Psychological inciters
(1) Attractive partner
(2) Erotic stimulation
(3) Fantasy
(4) Love
(5) Courtship

Sexual suppressors

Physiologic suppressors
(1) Hormone disorders
(2) Drug with sexual side-effects
(3) Depression

Psychological inhibitors
(1) Unattractive partner
(2) Negative thoughts
(3) Anti-fantasies
(4) Negative emotions
(5) Stress and anger

Hypothalamic and limbic sex-regulating centers

+   −

Sexual desire

Subjective experience of lust

Sexual avoidance

Prior to 1980, sexual dysfunction of any cause was lumped under the term 'impotence' for men and 'frigidity' for women. Since then, the classification of sexual disorders has been based on the physiologically oriented, four-phase model of human sexuality (Chapter 14). This classification divides the sexual dysfunction syndromes into disorders of desire, excitement/arousal and orgasm; the fourth phase of the human sexual response, resolution, is rarely disturbed. Sexual desire disorders include hyper- and hypoactive sexual drive (libido) and sexual aversion. Excitement phase disorders include erectile dysfunction, dyspareunia and vagnismus. Orgasmic disorders include inhibited orgasm in women and premature ejaculation in men.

Sexual desire disorders

Normal sexual drive can be thought of as a balance between an 'erotic motor' which incites a desire for sexual activity and a 'sexual brake' which keeps these urges in check so that we do not court disaster. These excitatory and inhibitory signals appear to converge upon specific centres in the hypothalamus and limbic system to produce a continuum of sexual desire of which only the polar ends are probably abnormal. Even given these guidelines, there is no specific test for abnormal sexual desire. Instead, the diagnosis of a sexual desire disorder is based on the subjective reporting of abnormal libido that results in individual distress or interpersonal difficulty.

The two formally recognized sexual desire disorders are hypoactive sexual disorder (HSD) and sexual aversion disorder. HSD is defined as persistently or recurrently deficient (or absent) sexual fantasies and desire for sexual activity. Sexual aversion disorder is the persistent or recurrent extreme aversion to, and avoidance of, all (or almost all) genital sexual contact with a sexual partner. Of patients seeking treatment for sexual desire disorders, 79% have HSD, 20% have sexual aversion disorder and 1% have hyperactive sexual desires. The causes of sexual desire disorders may be either organic or psychosocial. Organic causes include testosterone deficiency, chronic illness, certain centrally acting medications and underlying psychiatric disturbances. Psychogenic causes include psychologically repressive stimuli such as perception of a partner as repulsive, anxiety, anger or previous negative experiences.

Treatment of the sexual desire disorders is directed toward evaluation and correction of any underlying organic problem, and psychotherapy.

Erectile dysfunction (impotence)

Many men cannot get an erection from time to time and this is normal. Erectile dysfunction (ED) is the inability of a man to get and keep an erection sufficient for intercourse on multiple occasions. ED is mild if a man can usually get and keep an erection, moderate if only sometimes he can get or keep an erection and complete if he never can. Risk factors for ED including aging, chronic illnesses, various medications and cigarette smoking. It is a pervasive problem among older men; recent estimates are that 50% of 40–70-year-old men have some degree of ED and even more after age 70.

ED can occur because of vasculogenic, neurogenic, hormonal or psychogenic problems. Eighty per cent of the diagnosable conditions leading to ED are organic. They include in order of frequency: atherosclerosis, diabetes, hypertension, medication side-effects, prostate surgery, hyper- and hypothyroidism, hyperprolactinemia and hypogonadism. Depression is present in 60% of men with ED, but whether it is the cause or result of the disorder is often unclear.

Successful penile erection involves autonomic nerve activity on the vascular smooth muscle of the penis such that blood flows in to the penis and is trapped there (Chapter 12). Most of the organic causes of ED involve neuropathies of the autonomic nervous system, vascular compromise or occasionally, testosterone deficiency. Psychogenic ED involves abnormal central inhibition of the erectile mechanism without any demonstrable physical abnormality. Drugs that produce ED are myriad and typically affect the neural reflex pathways necessary for integrating the erection. Examples of medications associated with ED are antidepressants, antipsychotics, sedatives, antianxiety medications, antihypertensives and anticonvulsants. Alcohol and street drugs including amphetamines, cocaine, marijuana, methadone and heroin can also cause ED.

Until recently, treatment options for ED were limited to medication changes, implantable erection devices, intracavernosal injections of prostaglandins and psychotherapy. The discovery that the drug sildenafil can facilitate and maintain erections in impotent men has changed the treatment of ED dramatically. Sildenafil was originally tried as an antiangina medication and found to be ineffective. The study subjects were reluctant to turn in their leftover pills and soon the drug's unexpected side-effect was uncovered. Since then sildenafil, which is marketed under the tradename Viagra, has been tested in multiple clinical trials and is widely available for the treatment of ED. Sildenafil works by inhibiting PDE5, a nitric oxide metabolizing enzyme mainly found in the penis. Nitric oxide (NO) is the major mediator of the vascular relaxation necessary for penile erection and the longer NO stays around, the longer the erection. Unlike the implantable erection devices, sildenafil does not cause erections in the absence of sexual stimuli.

Premature ejaculation

Premature ejaculation is a disorder characterized by recurrent ejaculations with minimal sexual stimulation after penetration and before the man wishes it. When making the diagnosis, the man's age, the novelty of the sexual partner and circumstances and his frequency of sexual activity must be taken into account. Premature ejaculation is reported by 10–35% of men seeking help for sexual dysfunction. Unlike ED, which increases with age, premature ejaculation decreases with age.

The exact cause of premature ejaculation is unknown. The only demonstrable physiologic correlate of premature ejaculation is that men reporting this disorder ejaculate at a lower level of sexual arousal than do control men.

Retrograde ejaculation

Retrograde ejaculation occurs when the semen travels backwards into the bladder rather than out of the penile shaft during ejaculation. It occurs when the bladder neck does not close following emission. Like ED, retrograde ejaculation occurs as a result of an organic problem that is almost always neurologic in origin. The three most common causes of retrograde ejaculation are prostate surgery that affects penile innervation, diabetic neuropathy and anticholinergic medications. Retrograde ejaculation does not require intervention unless a pregnancy is desired.

Dyspareunia

Dyspareunia is the presence of recurrent or persistent genital pain in either a male or female before, during or after sexual intercourse. Most commonly, the pain is experienced during intercourse. Between 10 and 30% of women seeking help with sexual problems report dyspareunia while only 1% of men report the problem. Because dyspareunia is reported so much more frequently in women than in men, much more is known about it in women.

Dyspareunia may reflect a physical or psychogenic problem. Details of whether the symptoms are lifelong or acquired, generalized or situational are helpful in identifying the potential etiology. Organic causes of dyspareunia include hymeneal remnants, pelvic tumors, endometriosis, pelvic inflammatory disease, vulvar vestibulitis and hypoestrogenic states such as very low dose oral contraceptive use, menopause, early postpartum period and after chemotherapy. Psychosocial problems may revolve around the woman herself and include poor self-esteem, poor body image, guilt and prior sexual abuse or trauma. Interpersonal factors within the couple, including anger, distrust and inadequate communication may be responsible.

Treatment of dyspareunia is directed toward evaluation and correction of any underlying organic problem, and psychotherapy.

Vaginismus

Vaginismus is the recurrent occurrence of involuntary spasms of the pelvic muscles located in the outer third of the vaginal barrel such that they interfere with intercourse. Typically the muscle spasms occur in anticipation of intercourse or during penetration; however, they can also occur during a pelvic examination or tampon insertion in extreme cases.

Vaginismus occurs in 0.5–5% of women, with significant intercultural differences. Lifelong vaginismus is a rare clinical entity in North America and most of Western Europe. It is relatively common in Ireland, Eastern Europe and Latin America. It is the most commonly reported cause of unconsummated marriages.

Like dyspareunia, vaginismus can have either an organic or psychosocial etiology. The organic bases of the disorder are the same as dyspareunia. Most experts believe that vaginismus begins as dyspareunia and escalates to vaginismus through a classical conditioning process. Thus a woman has pain on intercourse (unconditioned stimulus), which leads to a natural self-protecting tightening of the vaginal muscles (conditioned response). Over time, stimuli associated with vaginal penetration, including thoughts of sexual intercourse, can become conditioned stimuli and provoke the conditioned reflex muscle spasms.

Not all cases of vaginismus are classically conditioned from an organic cause. Many psychosocial contributors have been suggested including guilt, religious constraints, responses to a partner's sexual dysfunction, prior sexual trauma, concerns about sexual orientation and fears of pregnancy, sexually transmitted diseases and trauma.

Like dyspareunia, treatment of vaginismus is directed toward evaluation and correction of any underlying organic problem, and psychotherapy.

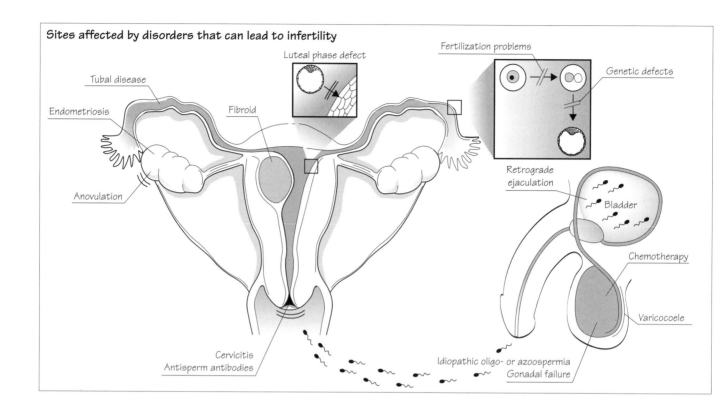

Sites affected by disorders that can lead to infertility

Infertility is defined as a diminished capacity to conceive and bear a child. It is not the same as sterility, which is the absolute and irreversible inability to conceive. Clinically, a couple is considered infertile if they are unable to conceive after 12 months of unprotected, frequent coitus. It is estimated that 10–15% of married couples in the United States are infertile.

There are many factors that contribute to infertility. Diseases that affect the female partner account for about one-third of infertile couples, diseases that affect the male only, about 10% of infertile couples and in another third of couples, both partners have abnormalities. About 20% of couples have no identifiable cause for their infertility or become pregnant during the evaluation. The disorders that are associated with infertility include those that involve each of the major physiologic events that are necessary to produce a pregnancy. These include: (i) production of a healthy egg; (ii) production of healthy sperm; (iii) transportation of the sperm to the site of fertilization and transportation of the zygote to the uterus for implantation; (iv) successful implantation in a receptive endometrium; and (v) presence of other conditions, often immunological, that can interfere with any one or more of the other necessary events.

Oocyte abnormalities

By far the most common oocyte abnormality is failure to ovulate. The same disorders that cause anovulation can produce amenorrhea and are covered in detail in Chapter 28. The disorders can be grouped into three general categories: hypothalamic dysfunction, pituitary disease and ovarian dysfunction.

Common hypothalamic causes of anovulation include abnormalities of weight and body composition, strenuous exercise, stress and travel. Pituitary or endocrine disorders that are often associated with anovulation are hyperprolactinemia and hypothyroidism. The two most common causes of ovarian dysfunction are polycystic ovary syndrome and premature ovarian failure. Oocyte abnormalities that are more complex than simple anovulation are responsible for the decline in fertility that occurs as women enter their 40s.

Female anatomic abnormalities

Tubal disease is usually the result of inflammatory scarring of the Fallopian tubes from pelvic inflammatory disease, appendicitis with rupture, septic abortion, previous surgery and previous use of an intrauterine device. Pelvic adhesions that compromise or destroy the fimbriated end of the tube are most often encountered and may affect as many as 20% of the women in infertile couples.

Endometriosis is a common disorder characterized by the presence of tissue that resembles endometrium outside of its normal position lining the uterus. The glands and stroma of endometriosis are usually responsive to gonadal hormones and the biochemical changes the steroids induce in the ectopic endometrium mimic those seen in perimenstrual endometrium. Increased prostaglandin production is thought to promote the inflammation, fibrosis and adhesion formation characteristic of the disorder. Endometriosis lesions can be found almost anywhere in the pelvis but are most common on the peritoneal surfaces covering the pouch of Douglas, the bladder, the ovaries, the Fallopian tubes, the bowel and the appendix. Women with endometriosis can present with pelvic pain, an adnexal mass (endometrioma) or infertility.

Uterine **leiomyomas**, also known as fibroids or uterine myomas, are benign smooth muscle tumors of the uterus. They are the most common pelvic tumor in women. Leiomyomas may be located anywhere in the wall of the uterus or hanging off a stalk containing the blood supply to the tumor. Only leiomyomas that distort the uterine cavity (submucosal in location) appear associated with decreased fecundity.

Male factors

A **varicocele** is a dilatation of the pampiniform plexus of veins that drain the scrotum. Varicoceles appear to reduce semen quality in some men either by increasing testicular temperature or by exposing the testis to abnormally high concentrations of an inhibitor of sperm function because of decreased venous efflux.

Blockage of the vas deferens or epididymis can either be a congenital abnormality caused by mutations in the cystic fibrosis transmembrane regulator gene (Chapter 24) or be caused by inadvertent surgical ligation at the time of inguinal surgery.

Retrograde ejaculation is caused by damage to the bladder neck or by injury to the lumbar sympathetic nerves involved in the ejaculation reflex. Sperm end up back in the bladder instead of the ejaculate and may be harvested from the urine if medical therapy is not effective.

Men may also produce very few or no sperm because of inadequate stimulation of the testis from either hypogonadotropic hypogonadism (Kallman syndrome) or gonadal failure such as is seen with Klinefelter syndrome (47,XXY). Occasionally no cause can be found. Men with oligospermia from Kallman syndrome are the best candidates for treatment with gonadotropins; the others do not respond.

Implantation abnormalities

Luteal phase deficiency, which is actually an ovarian problem, appears to reduce fertility by delaying maturation of the endometrium. In luteal phase deficiency, abnormal follicular development and ovulation leads to a relative deficiency in progesterone production. This then delays or minimizes the effects of progesterone in converting the endometrium into a secretory organ receptive to implantation. It appears as if the endometrial maturation must lag by 4 days or more for fecundity to be reduced.

Other factors

Miscellaneous other factors can influence fecundity, notably a group of immunological factors. Antisperm antibodies have been identified in some patients with infertility but have also been detected in fertile couples. Inflammatory cells recruited into cervical mucus as a result of cervical infections may affect sperm function, perhaps through release of cytokines. Some women develop antibodies against negatively charged phospholipids commonly encountered in cell membranes. These antiphospholipid antibodies can cause thromboses in small vessels leading to local ischemia and infarction. Although antiphospholipid antibodies more typically result in recurrent early miscarriage, some women experience loss so early as not to know they are even pregnant.

Genetic abnormalities such as the androgen insensitivity (Chapter 24) and gonadal dysgenesis syndromes (Chapters 24 and 25) can also cause infertility.

Evaluation and treatment of infertility

Evaluation of the infertile couple involves assessment of the male partner with a semen analysis, assessment of ovarian reserve by the measurement of FSH and estradiol in the early follicular phase of the cycle, anatomic assessment of the uterine cavity and fallopian tube patency with a hysterosalpingogram (HSG) and, when indicated, a laparoscopy or hysteroscopy.

Once the evaluation is complete, treatment of the infertile couple is directed by the findings. Women who are anovulatory or oligo-ovulatory are treated either by correction of any underlying problem such as hyperprolactinemia or hypothyroidism or by induction of ovulation with clomiphene citrate or gonadotropin injections.

Reproductive tract surgery to remove endometriosis or a fibroid tumor may be recommended although medical therapy for some of these problems is also available. In the past, tubal reconstructive surgery was a mainstay of infertility treatment; *in vitro* fertilization (IVF) has virtually eliminated the need for this approach.

Male factor infertility can also be approached by either correcting the underlying problem such as a varicocoele or by using IVF techniques designed to bypass sperm problems. In some cases, artificial insemination of the woman with her husband's or a donor's sperm may be chosen.

The widespread availability of the assisted reproductive technologies has revolutionized the treatment of infertility, making pregnancies possible under circumstances never before considered treatable. The options now available include gamete intrafallopian transfer (GIFT), zygote intrafallopian transfer (ZIFT) and *in vitro* fertilization (IVF). In GIFT and ZIFT, the egg and sperm or embryo, respectively, are transferred to the Fallopian tube of the woman. In IVF, multiple harvested eggs are fertilized by spermatozoa in the laboratory and 2–3-day-old embryos are transferred back into the women's uterus. IVF can be modified to use donor eggs or donor sperm and even to inject a single sperm into the cytoplasm of an egg to overcome severe male factor infertility (intracytoplasmic sperm injection; ICSI).

33 Multifetal pregnancy

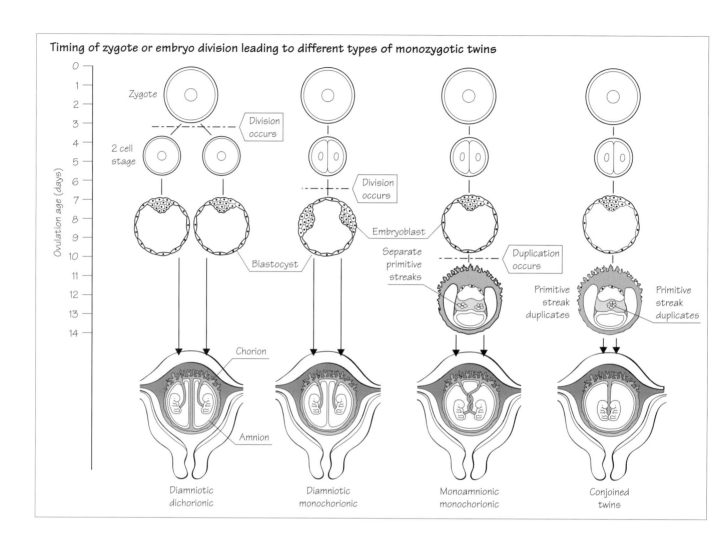

Timing of zygote or embryo division leading to different types of monozygotic twins

Ovulation age (days)

Zygote

2 cell stage

Division occurs

Division occurs

Blastocyst

Embryoblast

Separate primitive streaks

Duplication occurs

Primitive streak duplicates

Primitive streak duplicates

Chorion

Amnion

| Diamniotic dichorionic | Diamniotic monochorionic | Monoamnionic monochorionic | Conjoined twins |

Overview

Twins may arise from one of two mechanisms, division of a single fertilized ovum into two embryos (**'identical' or monozygotic twins**) or fertilization of two separate ova (**'fraternal' or dizygotic twins**). Either or both processes may be involved in the generation of higher numbers of fetuses. Triplets could develop from one, two or three ova; quadruplets from one, two, three or four and so on. It is rare, however, for a zygote to divide more than once.

The biology of the two twinning processes is quite different in both origin and implication for the pregnancy outcome. While all multiple gestations carry a risk of preterm delivery from early labor, monozygotic twin pregnancies carry an additional risk of placental problems, chromosomal abnormalities and malformations that can dramatically influence the pregnancy outcome.

Biology of monozygotic twinning

The exact mechanism by which an embryo is stimulated to divide to produce monozygotic twins is not known. It is clear from studies of the relationships of the extrafetal tissues (membranes and placentas) and

from the genetic identity of the fetuses that division of the fertilized ovum at specific early stages of development is responsible for the spectrum of monozygotic twinning. These stages are depicted in the figure above. Basically, the earlier the division, the more separate the twins, i.e. cleavage prior to development of an inner cell mass will result in two placentas, two sets of membranes and two fetuses whereas division after an embryonic disk has formed results in conjoined twins.

The most common type of monozygotic twins arises from division between the 3rd and 8th day after fertilization. This produces a pregnancy with two amniotic sacs and a single placenta (**diamniotic monochorionic twins**). The second most common type of monozygotic twinning results from a division of the embryo within the first 72 h after fertilization and produces two amniotic sacs and two placentas (**diamniotic dichorionic twins**). Fraternal twins are always diamniotic dichorionic so that it is necessary to do zygosity testing on twins with separate placentas who are suspected of being monozygous. Twins resulting from divisions later than day 8 after fertilization are rare. If the division occurs on or after day 8 when the amnion forms, both fetuses will be in the same amniotic sac (**monoamniotic monochorionic** twins). Siamese or **conjoined twins** are the rarest and arise between days 13 and 16 post conception from cleavage of the differentiating embryonic disk.

Etiology of dizygotic twins

Most spontaneously conceived multifetal pregnancies are twin gestations. The incidence of conception of twins is at least twice the rate of liveborn twins. In many cases, one of a pair of diamniotic dichorionic twins just disappears. Less often, the whole pregnancy miscarries. The frequency of monozygotic twinning is about 1 set in every 250 births and is relatively fixed in most populations. In contrast to monozygotic twinning, the incidence of dizygotic twinning is quite varied in different populations. Dizygotic twinning is highly influenced by race, maternal age over 40, parity, heredity and infertility treatment.

The racial differences in dyzygotic twinning are quite marked. Twinning among Asians is least common, with a rate of only 1.3 dizygotic twin births per 1000 total births in Japan. White women in the United States and the United Kingdom have rates of about 8 dizygotic twin sets per 1000 births. Black women have the highest rates of all. They range from a rate of 11 per 1000 births in the United States to 49 per 1000 in some tribes in Nigeria, or 1 in every 20 births! The influence of heredity is carried largely through maternal lineages, with about a 2% chance of delivering twins if the mother herself is a dizygotic twin. When the father of the baby is a dizygotic twin, the rate of twinning is only 0.8%.

Most multifetal pregnancies now conceived in developed countries are the result of infertility treatment. Ovulation induction, gamete intrafallopian transfer (GIFT), zygote intrafallopian transfer (ZIFT) and *in vitro* fertilization (IVF) all dramatically increase the frequency not only of twinning, but of conceiving higher order multiple gestations, that is, triplets, quadruplets and more. The table below lists the approximate frequency of multifetal pregnancies in the 1990s in the United States, dependent on the means of conception. If one uses Hellin's theorem to calculate the expected frequency of twins in Nigeria, which has the highest spontaneous twinning rate in the world, one can see the impact of infertility treatment on the higher order gestations. Hellin's theorum states that if the frequency of twinning is n in a population, then the frequency of triplets is n^2, quadruplets n^3, and so on. Using $n = 0.05$ for the Nigerian tribes, one would only expect 0.25% triplet and 0.012% quadruplet gestations. Thus infertility treatment increases the risk of triplets 20-fold and quadruplets 80-fold over the world's most 'twinningest' people!

Multifetal pregnancy rates using different infertility treatments (% of births).

Treatment	Twins	Triplets	Quadruplets+
None	1.2	0.015	0.00017
Clomiphene	8–10	<1	–
Gonadotropins	15	5	0.6
GIFT, ZIFT, IVF	28	6	1

GIFT, gamete intrafallopian transfer; IVF, *in vitro* fertilization; ZIFT, zygote intrafallopian transfer.

Although infertility treatment dramatically increases the frequency of non-identical multiples, the rate of monozygous twins is also about double that expected in these women. A disproportionate number of these monozygotic twins are also monochorionic. The stimulus for monozygotic twinning following ovulation induction has not been identified.

It is generally agreed that the single largest risk factor for dizygotic conceptions is elevated gonadotropin levels in the conception cycle. Elevated gonadotropins appear to increase recruitment of more than one ovarian follicle in the conception cycle. This is most evident during infertility treatments where the use of injected gonadotropins is associated with multiple ovulatory follicles seen on ultrasound of the ovaries. Elevated endogenous gonadotropins, notably FSH, appear also to explain the increased rates of spontaneous twinning seen with black race, advancing maternal age, parity and heredity.

Pregnancy risks with multiples

The relationships of the placenta and fetal membranes play a distinct role in the risk of subsequent problems in a multifetal pregnancy. All monochorionic twins have vascular connections within the placental bed. In about 20% of monochorionic twin pregnancies, these vascular connections permit exchange of blood between the two fetuses. The hemodynamics of the two twins can become so deranged that one fetus is preferentially pumping extra blood into the other (the so-called **'twin–twin transfusion syndrome'**). The 'donor' twin becomes anemic and has abnormally low amniotic fluid in its sac whereas the 'recipient' twin is volume overloaded and has an excess of amniotic fluid in its sac. Multiple gestations also have an increased risk of abnormal umbilical cord insertions onto their placentas. Usually the umbilical cord inserts in the middle of the placental disk and is surrounded completely by a protective layer of Warton's jelly. Multiple fetuses have an increased incidence of cord insertions on the edge of the placenta that are not completely surrounded by Warton's jelly (**velamentous insertion**). Cords with velamentous insertions can be kinked or compressed more readily, thereby leading to suboptimal blood flow into that fetus. Monoamniotic twins always have their umbilical cords entangled, leading to fetal deaths in over half of the cases.

In addition to the problems that can arise from their placentas and membranes, monozygotic twins are also at increased risk of chromosomal abnormalities and congenital malformations. Because affected twin pairs are often discordant for the abnormality, it is presumed that whatever intrauterine events cause embryos to divide also randomly increase the risk for disordered embryonic development.

All multiple gestations are also at risk for growth restriction of one or more of the fetuses (Chapter 34.4). The risk increases as the number of fetuses increases. The causes of the growth restriction can be suboptimal perfusion in the area of placental implantation of one or more fetus, decreased fetal perfusion from a velamentous umbilical cord insertion or the donation of blood to a cotwin in the twin–twin transfusion syndrome.

All multiple gestations are at risk for preterm labor (Chapter 34, section 3). The risk increases with increasing numbers of fetuses. One potential mechanism for the early onset of labor is uterine distension; however, other non-mechanical factors may also be involved.

34 Pregnancy complications

1 EARLY PREGNANCY LOSS

Miscarriage

A miscarriage is defined as a spontaneous pregnancy loss before 20 weeks of gestation. The medical term for miscarriage is **spontaneous abortion**. Miscarriages occur in 15% of recognized pregnancies. The total number of human conceptions far exceeds the number of births. It is estimated that at least 60% of all human conceptions do not result in a viable pregnancy. The majority of these conceptions are spontaneously lost before or shortly after an expected menses, as documented by the appearance and disappearance of pregnancy hormone (hCG; Chapter 17) from the maternal bloodstream. It is clear that there is a sensitive and effective system for detecting abnormal pregnancies and not permitting the vast majority to continue.

It is impossible to know what the causes are of those pregnancy losses that occur shortly around the expected menses, the so-called 'chemical pregnancies'. They are probably due to a myriad of abnormalities in both the conceptus and the endocrine microenvironment of the maternal reproductive tract at the time of conception. It is known that the most frequent cause of overt miscarriage is a chromosomal abnormality in the conceptus. At least 60% of miscarriages have a gross chromosomal abnormality detectable in the expelled fetal material. The table below lists the frequency with which specific chromosomal abnormalities are identified in miscarried material. It is usually not possible to identify a cause for the remaining 40% of miscarriages, although a small number are the result of an underlying problem that can lead to recurrent miscarriages (see below).

The frequency of both chromosomal abnormal and abnormal miscarriage is age dependent, as may be seen in the figure at the top of the page. The dramatic rise in miscarriage after maternal age 35 is thought to be due to aging problems in the egg. Ovum deterioration is thought to explain most of the decline in fertility after age 40 as well.

Bleeding in the first trimester and a fall in hCG herald most miscarriages. During the first 12 weeks of pregnancy, hCG normally rises

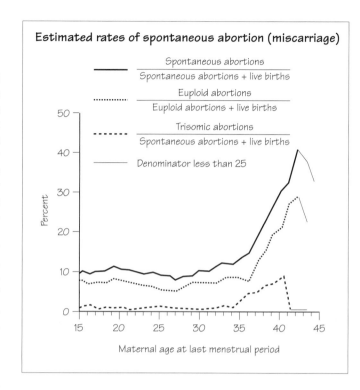

Relative frequency of aberrations in chromosomally abnormal abortuses.

Type	Incidence (%)
Trisomy	(52 total trisomy)
14	3.7
15	4.2
16	16.4
18	3.0
21	4.7
22	5.7
Other	14.3
45,X	18
Triploid	17
Tetraploid	6
Unbalanced translocation	3
Other	4
Total	100

with a doubling time of about 48–72 h. Threatened miscarriages will show a plateau or drop in hCG before tissue is passed. Thus, it would appear that the common signaling mechanism for abnormal pregnancies is a disruption in the expression of the hCG gene located on chromosome 19. How trisomies and other chromosomal aneuploidies produce this effect on the hCG gene is not known. It is equally puzzling how the three trisomies that can be carried to viability, trisomies 13, 18 and 21, escape the surveillance. Trisomy 21 is actually associated with an increase in circulating hCG in the second trimester; this finding is used as part of triple serum screening for Down syndrome risk.

Recurrent miscarriage

Because one in every six pregnancies will result in a miscarriage, it is not uncommon for a woman to experience one or more during her pregnancy attempts. Once a woman has had three consecutive miscarriages, however, the odds increase that it is not just a random event but related to an underlying recurrent problem.

Causes of recurrent miscarriage (habitual abortion) include parental chromosome translocations; structural uterine abnormalities such as longitudinal septa and intrauterine adhesions; endocrine disorders including luteal phase defects, polycystic ovary syndrome (PCOS), hyperprolactinemia, thyroid dysfunction and poorly controlled diabetes mellitus; infections with mycoplasma and ureaplasma; and autoimmune conditions, notably the antiphospholipid antibody syndrome. Couples experiencing recurrent pregnancy losses are appropriately anxious and should be evaluated for an underlying cause in the hope that something can be done to prevent another miscarriage.

2 DIABETES

Maternal glucose regulation in pregnancy

Pregnancy requires that a steady stream of nutrients be available to the growing fetus, especially in the last third of pregnancy when fetal growth may exceed an ounce (28 g) a day. One of the primary fetal fuels is glucose. The placenta has an abundance of glucose transporters, thereby permitting glucose transport at a rate that is limited only by the maternal supply. Maternal metabolism is thus altered to reduce glucose uptake by maternal cells in order to ensure an adequate supply for the fetus.

The main mechanism by which maternal metabolism is altered is by increasing peripheral insulin resistance. Although the placenta produces several hormones which can affect insulin secretion or activity, **human placental lactogen** (hPL); also known as **chorionic somatomammotropin (hCS)**, is likely responsible for most of the peripheral insulin resistance. The effects of hPL on fat and carbohydrate metabolism are similar to those seen with GH and include inhibition of peripheral glucose uptake, stimulation of insulin release by the pancreas and an increase in plasma free fatty acids (Chapter 17). Once cellular uptake of glucose is impeded, transient maternal hyperglycemia occurs after meals. This increment in circulating glucose is then available to the fetus but also causes additional insulin secretion by the mother. Circulating glucose levels drop as a consequence of both fetal uptake and movement into the maternal cells so that, between meals, most pregnant women are relatively hypoglycemic. After a period of fasting, such as overnight, hPL promotes lipolysis. Fats and ketones derived from the circulating lipids are an additional source of fuel to the fetus.

Gestational diabetes

About 3–4% of otherwise normal pregnant women cannot increase their pancreatic production of insulin sufficiently to overcome the insulin resistance and maintain euglycemia. Such a condition is known as gestational diabetes mellitus (GDM). It resembles type II diabetes very closely in that peripheral insulin resistance and pancreatic insufficiency underlie both disorders. Gestational diabetes and type II diabetes are so closely linked that glucose intolerance in pregnancy is one of the best screening tests available for lifetime risk of developing type II diabetes. Over 50% of women diagnosed with GDM in any pregnancy will develop type II diabetes within 20 years of that pregnancy. Risk factors for developing GDM include a family history of type II diabetes, obesity, advancing maternal age, native American race and previous history of GDM.

GDM typically develops in the latter part of pregnancy when placental hPL secretion is maximal and so is insulin resistance. The major complication of untreated GDM is fetal overgrowth. Fetal overgrowth from diabetes develops because of fetal hyperinsulinemia. When maternal glucose levels remain abnormally high, fetal glucose will also be high. The fetus, which is not exposed to the same high levels of hPL that the mother is, secretes insulin appropriately to lower blood sugar. The hyperinsulinemia that develops favors fuel storage as fat. Fetal insulin-like growth factors I and II (IGF-I and IGF-II) are also elevated in diabetic pregnancies. The IGFs are involved in somatic growth of the skeleton and organs and are likely responsible for the overall increase in size of infants of diabetic mothers.

Fetal overgrowth is a clinical problem because of birth injuries that can accompany delivery of excessively large infants. Large or macrosomic infants of diabetic mothers are at increased risk of birth injury over comparably sized infants of non-diabetics because of truncal fat deposition. Head size is increased only minimally and the head delivers normally. The shoulders and trunk can then become stuck in the birth canal, leading to birth asphyxia and brachial plexus injuries. Fetal overgrowth can be minimized, but not eliminated entirely, by tight glycemic control with diet and insulin when necessary. Maternal obesity, which is an independent risk factor for fetal macrosomia, compounds the risk of fetal overgrowth in diabetic women.

Pregestational diabetes

Pregestational diabetes complicates about 0.5% of all pregnancies. The presence of hyperglycemia during embryogenesis carries with it the risks of congenital anomalies and miscarriage in addition to the common problem of fetal overgrowth. Diabetic embryopathy is uncommon, but still possible, with tight blood sugar control surrounding conception. The risk increases dramatically with poor control such that rates of anomalies and miscarriage are threefold higher in patients with the poorest control. The most common anomalies are neural tube and cardiac defects.

The mechanisms by which hyperglycemia disturbs embryonic development are not yet completely elucidated. The types and severity of the anomalies suggest that the embryopathy develops at the yolk sac stage, which is 6–7 weeks after fertilization. Excess free radical production resulting from glucose-initiated cellular hypermetabolism appears to be involved, as antioxidants and free radical scavengers can inhibit hyperglycemic-induced embryopathy in an animal model. There also appears to be a genetic component that determines both susceptibility and organ specificity to the ensuing damage. The increased miscarriage rate with poor glycemic control early in pregnancy is probably related to embryopathy incompatible with survival.

Infants of diabetic mothers

Infants of diabetic mothers suffer from a number of problems directly related to maternal hyperglycemia. In addition to the risk of congenital anomalies and birth injury from fetal overgrowth, these infants are at risk for respiratory distress, profound hypoglycemia, polycythemia, hyperbilirubinemia and hypocalcemia. The respiratory distress results from a negative impact of diabetes upon fetal surfactant production. Profound hypoglycemia can occur when the maternal source of glucose is interrupted at birth in a hyperinsulinemic fetus. Polycythemia develops as compensation when persistent maternal hyperglycemia leads to increased oxygen demands within the fetoplacental unit. Hyperbilirubinemia results when the increased red cell mass of the polycythemic newborn begins to break down before the baby's immature liver can handle the load. In addition, the abnormalities of growth and metabolism encountered *in utero* from maternal diabetes can extend into later life as well. Glucose intolerance, obesity and hypertension are increased among older children and adults whose mothers had diabetes.

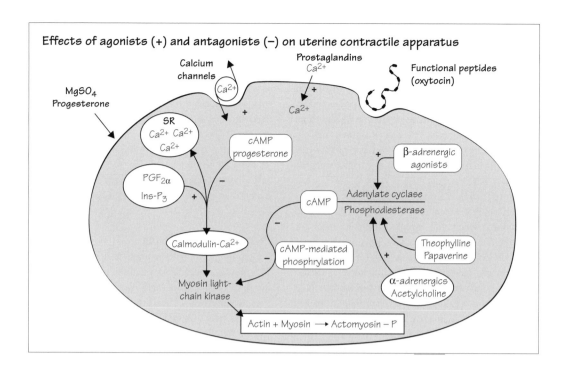

Effects of agonists (+) and antagonists (−) on uterine contractile apparatus

3 PRETERM LABOR

Overview

Preterm labor is the onset of labor before 37 weeks of gestation. It is the final common pathway for a number of conditions that induce uterine contractions at a time when the uterus is normally quiescent.

Preterm labor complicates 7–10% of all pregnancies and is a very large contributor to perinatal morbidity and mortality. Although over half the cases of preterm labor occur without warning, some factors do carry an identifiable risk. These include multiple gestation, uterine anomalies, third trimester bleeding, intrauterine infection, excessive amniotic fluid volume, smoking and a history of prior preterm delivery. There have been numerous unsuccessful attempts to predict women at high risk for preterm labor. To date, strategies that have not worked well are risk scoring, close clinical observation and home uterine contraction monitoring. Several biochemical markers suggest increased risk of preterm labor. These include increases in salivary estriol, which reflects activation of the fetal hypothalamic–pituitary–adrenal axis; cortisol-releasing hormone, which is synthesized by the placenta (Chapter 19); and relaxin, a decidual hormone. Fetal fibronectin, which normally is restricted to the fetal compartment, appears in vaginal secretions in women who are at risk for preterm delivery. More importantly, its absence is highly predictive of women who will not have preterm labor.

Potential mechanisms for preterm labor

The pathways by which some stimuli start labor prematurely may be deduced from knowledge of the normal mechanisms involved in labor (Chapter 19). For instance, intrauterine infection is associated with an elevation in the cytokines interleukin-1β, interleukin-6 and tumor necrosis factor α (TNF-α) in the amniotic fluid. Products of both the cyclooxygenase and prostaglandin pathways are also elevated in patients with intrauterine infections. Cytokines and prostaglandins act synergistically in stimulating the myometrium and could activate the uterus prematurely. Recently, thrombin has been shown to be an extremely potent uterotonic agent and is probably responsible for the preterm labor associated with bleeding in pregnancy. Another group of patients appears to have a deficiency in the enzyme 15-hydroxyprostaglandin dehydrogenase that is normally present in large amounts in the placenta and deciduas. This enzyme is responsible for degrading some of the prostaglandins stimulatory to labor. Multiple gestations and excessive amniotic fluid both invoke overstretching of the myometrial syncytium, but how this actually produces the regular, coordinated contractions of labor is unknown.

Pharmacologic interventions

In some cases of preterm labor, the contractions represent the attempt by the uterus to expel the fetus from a hostile intrauterine environment such as an intrauterine infection. Whenever this appears to be happening, it is wise not to intervene. If the fetus is not in danger, then pharmacologic attempts to stop the premature contractions may be used. Several agents, known as **tocolytics**, are available. Tocolytics work by interrupting one of three processes: (i) intracellular calcium homeostasis; (ii) prostaglandin synthesis; or (iii) oxytocin binding to its receptors (see diagram above). Magnesium sulfate ($MgSO_4$), the most widely used tocolytic, works as a competitive antagonist for calcium needed for myometrial contractions. Nifedipine, a type II dipyridamole calcium channel blocker, prevents calcium influx through the cell membranes into the myometrial cells. β-Adrenergic agonists such as ritodrine, salbutamol, isoxuprine and terbutaline reduce intracellular calcium concentrations and decrease the sensitivity of the actin–myosin unit to calcium. Prostaglandins E and $F_{2\alpha}$ are stimulatory to uterine contractions. The tocolytic indometacin reduces prostaglandin production by inhibiting the cyclooxygenases necessary for conversion of arachidonic acid to prostaglandins. Oxytocin antagonists bind to the oxytocin receptor without activating it.

4 FETAL GROWTH RESTRICTION

Theoretically, fetal growth restriction (FGR) is present in any fetus that does not reach his/her growth potential. Practically speaking, it is usually restricted to those fetuses whose weight is less than the 10th percentile who also demonstrate other evidence of suboptimal growth, such as a decrease in their urine production (producing a secondary decrease in the amniotic fluid volume). It is important to identify fetuses with FGR because some of them are at risk of dying *in utero* and need to be carefully watched and delivered early whenever necessary. The causes of FGR can be divided into three general categories: fetal, maternal and uteroplacental.

Fetal causes of FGR

A fetal cause for FGR infers that something intrinsic to the fetus is interfering with fetal growth. Fetal causes for FGR include genetic factors, anomalies, multiple gestations and congenital infections. Mechanisms for the genetic causes are specific to underlying metabolic abnormalities. Most of the fetal anomalies that cause FGR do so by reducing blood flow to, or through, the fetus. Twins and higher-order multiples (triplets or more) typically affect each other's growth either by limiting placental perfusion due to crowding of the multiple placentae in the uterus, decreasing fetal perfusion when a velamentous cord insertion is present or by contributing to abnormal blood flow in the other twin through the placenta (twin–twin transfusion syndrome; Chapter 33). Congenital viral infections appear to cause FGR via cell death and dropout.

Maternal causes of FGR

Maternal causes of FGR include a number of maternal diseases and toxin/drug exposures. Almost anything that reduces maternal oxygen-carrying capacity can cause FGR. Most toxins and drugs that affect fetal growth do so by reducing blood flow through the uterus or placenta and could just as easily be characterized as uteroplacental factors. Antimetabolite chemotherapy probably reduces cell numbers, especially in the placenta, which remains a rapidly growing organ through most of pregnancy.

Uteroplacental causes of FGR

Uteroplacental factors are the most common cause of FGR. Either the uterine or the placental blood supply is compromised. Maternal hypertension, whether chronic or pregnancy induced, can reduce the blood flow into the uterine vascular lacunae underlying the placenta. Small blood clots, or microthrombi, can affect uteroplacental blood supply if they occur in either the uterine or placental vasculature. A compromise in blood flow in either the uterus or placenta then causes a progressive decline in growth. The mechanism by which fetal growth is reduced or stops is not simple starvation but appears to involve a decrease in fetal growth factors like the IGFs.

Most fetuses that die from FGR do so because perfusion is so poor that there is inadequate oxygen delivery to the fetus to sustain life any longer. These fetuses undergo a progressive deterioration in growth and well-being that begins with decreased body fat deposition. Next the growth of long bones slows. The growth of the head (brain) and other vital organs is initially spared but eventually their growth also slows.

Causes of fetal growth restriction.

Genetic factors
Chromosomal
  Trisomies (incidence of FGR; 18> 13>>21)
  Other
Single gene defects (e.g. dwarfism, maternal phenylketonuria)
Confined placental mosaicism

Fetal anomalies
Cardiovascular anomalies
Single umbilical artery
Bilateral renal agenesis
Velamentous insertion of the umbilical cord

Multiple gestation

Congenital infections
Rubella
Cytomegalovirus (CMV)
Human immunodeficiency virus (HIV)
Varicella

Drugs/toxins
Heavy cigarette smoking
Cocaine
Heroin
Coumarin
Phenytoin
Chemotherapy

Malnutrition
Maternal
  Gestational malnutrition in underweight women
  Cyanotic heart disease
  Chronic pulmonary disease
  Anemia
    Malaria
    Hemoglobinopathies
  Hyperthyroidism
Fetal
  Hyperthyroidism

Uteroplacental factors
Chronic hypertension
Pregnancy-induced hypertension
Antepartum placental abruption
Thrombophilia
  Inherited
    Protein S, C and antithrombin III deficiencies
    Factor V Leiden
    Prothrombin 2010
    Methylene tetrahydrofolate reductase deficiency
  Acquired
    Antiphospholipid antibodies
Unexplained chronic proteinuria
Previous FGR infant

The fetus can also become dehydrated so that it urinates so little that the amniotic fluid volume decreases. Finally, the fetus has so little oxygen available that it stops moving and dies shortly thereafter. Much clinical effort goes into trying to identify and deliver fetuses before they reach the end stages of FGR.

5 PREECLAMPSIA

Clinical spectrum of preeclampsia

Preeclampsia is a unique disorder that is found only in human pregnancies. **Historically preeclampsia has been defined as the triad of hypertension, proteinuria and edema** in a pregnant woman. Preeclampsia typically occurs in the third trimester of pregnancy, although some cases manifest earlier. **Eclampsia** is the occurence of seizures in a patient with preeclampsia that cannot be attributed to another cause. Although many patients with preeclampsia demonstrate this classic triad of hypertension, proteinuria and edema, it is now clear that the disorder is really a spectrum of clinical signs and symptoms that accompany microvascular changes in a number of organ systems. The disorder has so many presentations that some have called it the 'great imitator'. Central nervous system involvement can result in severe headaches, seizures, stroke, visual changes and blindness. Renal involvement is almost always present and can manifest as proteinuria, oliguria or renal failure. Hemoconcentration, thrombocytopenia and intravascular hemolysis are common signs of hematologic involvement. Edema can accumulate in many sites, including the feet, hands, face and lungs. Hepatic dysfunction often accompanies the hematologic changes and produces a syndrome known as **HELLP syndrome** (**h**emolysis, **e**levated **l**iver function tests, **l**ow **p**latelets). Patients with HELLP will often develop vague epigastric pain that is mistaken for heartburn, gallbladder disease or the flu by an unsuspecting general physician.

The overall incidence of preeclampsia in the obstetric population is 7–10%, depending on the proportion of patients at increased risk. Risk factors for developing preeclampsia include primigravida (first pregnancy), multiple gestation, diabetes, pre-existing hypertension, a new father in a multipara (one or more previous deliveries), history of preeclampsia in a previous pregnancy, inherited and acquired clotting disorders such as protein S and protein C deficiencies and antiphospholipid antibodies, and hydatidiform mole. There is considerable overlap in the risk factors for preeclampsia with those for fetal growth restriction (FGR). Indeed, the presence of FGR may be the first sign of impending preeclampsia and women with preeclampsia are at risk for delivering a growth-restricted baby.

Left untreated, preeclampsia can be a morbid and even fatal disease. The ultimate treatment is delivery; it is so effective a therapy that all the deranged physiology will revert to normal provided no permanent tissue damage has occurred. Thus, kidneys will begin to make urine again, blood will clot and seizures will stop provided that the mother is medically supported through a timely delivery and her postpartum recovery. In spite of its potential for a 100% cure with proper diagnosis and treatment, preeclampsia remains one of the leading causes of maternal death in both developed and developing countries.

Potential mechanisms in preeclampsia pathogenesis

The observation that delivery cures preeclampsia coupled with the increased risk for the disorder in patients with hydatidiform mole, a form of gestational trophoblast disease, pointed long ago to the placenta as the source of the problem. It was originally thought that the placenta secreted some substance, a toxin, that was responsible for the disorder and hence the old name 'toxemia'. While no toxins have been identified in the circulation of patients with preeclampsia, abnormal concentrations of specific metabolites are found in many of these patients. Circulating thromboxane, a vasoconstricting prostaglandin, is elevated while nitric oxide production is subnormal. Cytokines, placental fragments, and free radical and reactive oxygen species also have been found to be elevated in these patients. It is likely that the source of these abnormalities is a dysfunctional placenta.

Theories about what causes preeclampsia abound, but in truth we still do not know exactly what happens. There is some evidence for an immunological component to the disorder. Preeclampsia occurs most commonly in the first pregnancy but can occur for the first time in a later pregnancy if there is a different father of the baby. Failure to clear circulating immune complexes may be involved because of the similarities in symptoms between preeclampsia and other immune complex disorders (vasculitis, glomerular damage and activation of the clotting cascade). Immunological factors may also interfere with the normal invasion of the spiral arteries in the decidua, a common pathologic finding in the uterus of preeclamptic women. An immunological basis would explain the elevated cytokines in women with preeclampsia.

Other risk factors such as multiple gestation and maternal vascular disease suggest a mismatch between fetal/placental demands and the maternal ability to meet them as a pathogenetic mechanism in preeclampsia. Proponents of this theory propose that the fetus sends signals to the mother to increase perfusion of the placenta and, when the mother cannot compensate, excessive signal causes the disorder. Elevations in metabolites like thromboxane and free oxygen radicals support the fetal/placental mismatch theory.

Whatever the exact placental abnormality, the final pathway for preeclampsia is **endothelial dysfunction**. The normal function of the vascular endothelium is to prevent microcoagulation and to modulate vascular tone. Vascular injury results in coagulation and changes in the response of the underlying vascular smooth muscle to vasoactive substances. Often, substances that are vasodilators with an intact endothelium act as vasoconstrictors with a damaged endothelium. Thus, in preeclampsia, endothelial dysfunction can explain the basic triad: hypertension (vasospasm), edema (capillary leak) and proteinuria (renal cell damage secondary to hypoperfusion). Indeed all the protean signs and symptoms can be explained by endothelial dysfunction causing either vasospasm or microcoagulation. What remains inexplicable is why only a few, but not all, of the signs and symptoms appear in any one patient.

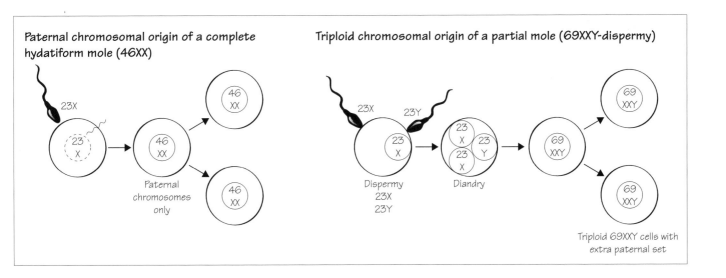

Paternal chromosomal origin of a complete hydatiform mole (46XX)

Triploid chromosomal origin of a partial mole (69XXY-dispermy)

Paternal chromosomes only

Dispermy 23X 23Y

Diandry

Triploid 69XXY cells with extra paternal set

6 GESTATIONAL TROPHOBLASTIC DISEASE

Gestational trophoblastic disease (GTD) is one of the earliest reported neoplasms. Hippocrates first described 'dropsy' of the uterus in 400 B.C. and a 13th century tombstone noted the birth of 365 'children', half boys and half girls, to the woman buried there. Today GTD retains its leading position in tumor biology as the most sensitive and curable of all human cancers. The genetic origin of molar pregnancies has also played a pivotal role in our understanding of the role of the maternal and paternal genome in embryonic development (Chapter 15).

There are a spectrum of diseases within the GTD classification: hydatidiform mole, either complete (CHM) or partial (PHM), persistent, non-metastatic GTD, metastatic good-prognosis GTD and metastatic poor-prognosis GTD which includes the histological tumors known as choriocarcinoma (CC). Of these, CHM and PHM follow abnormal conceptions and are restricted to women. Choriocarcinoma is unique among GTD in that it can arise from a normal conception, a molar pregnancy or a germ cell line. Choriocarcinoma in men is exclusively of germ-cell origin (Chapter 37).

Complete hydatidiform mole

Complete hydatidiform mole (CHM) is the most common of the GTDs and occurs in about 1/1000–1/1500 pregnancies in Western countries. It is at least twice as common in Asia and less common in black races. Extremes of age increase the risk for CHM, with women under age 15 and over age 40 at highest risk. Other risk factors include previous history of CHM, previous miscarriage, maternal balanced chromosomal translocation, professional occupation and perhaps a dietary deficiency of animal fat and carotene. A previously normal pregnancy lowers the risk of CHM.

CHM is characterized histologically by the presence of large amounts of hydropic villi without any fetal tissue. It presents clinically with delayed menses and the diagnosis of pregnancy. Pregnancy symptoms such as nausea and vomiting are often exaggerated because of the high chorionic gonadotropin (hCG) production by the abnormal trophoblast. Some patients with CHM will be hyperthyroid because of the stimulation of the thyroid gland by the hCG, which has some intrinsic thyroid-stimulating activity.

Treatment of CHM is evacuation of the molar tissue if fertility is to be preserved or hysterectomy if fertility is not to be preserved. Eighty per cent of CHMs will remit spontaneously; persistent disease requires chemotherapy for a cure. CHM is exquisitely sensitive to antimetabolite chemotherapy, typically methotrexate with folate rescue.

The unique genetic origins of CHM were suspected well before the advent of modern molecular techniques when karyotype analyses revealed that 96% of them were 46,XX. Polymerase chain reaction and restriction fragment length polymorphism (RFLP) analyses have demonstrated that **while CHM is always diploid, the chromosomes are all of paternal origin.** Most CHMs arise from fertilization of an enucleate, or empty egg, with a single 23,X sperm followed by duplication of the paternal haplotype. The remaining CHMs arise after fertilization of the enucleate egg with two sperm (dispermy); of these about one quarter, or 4% of the total CHMs, will have a 46,XY karyotype. All CHM has maternal mitochondrial DNA, confirming the contribution of the oocyte cell machinery; the mechanism by which the egg enucleates is not known. Degeneration of the chromosomes or extrusion of the female pronucleus with the polar body are two possibilities.

Partial hydatidiform mole

Partial hydatidiform mole (PHM) exists when proliferative villi with hydropic degeneration coexists with a fetus. Commonly the fetus dies by the late first or early second trimester and pathologic examination of the placenta is necessary to make the diagnosis because the hydropic villi are not as pronounced as they are in CHM. Patients with PHM tend to be older than those with CHM. PHM has a lower risk of subsequent malignancy than does CHM.

PHM pregnancies are all triploid with two copies of the paternal genome. PHM most commonly arises from dispermic fertilization (diandry) and occasionally from fertilization by a diploid sperm that failed to undergo a first or second reduction division during meiosis.

Persistent and metastatic gestational trophoblastic disease

Persistent and metastatic GTD are typically preceded by CHM and occasionally PHM or even normal pregnancies. Persistent GTD can invade the uterus or metastasize to liver, lung and brain, yet still has a very high cure rate with appropriate treatment.

Genetic study of neoplastic trophoblastic tissue is very important to the patient because gestational tumors have a better than 90% cure rate whereas non-gestational tumors with trophoblastic differentiation are essentially lethal.

35 Overview of neoplasia

In the purest sense, all cancers are genetic in origin in that they all are caused by DNA mutations. Any given tumor may arise from the accumulation of somatic mutations over time or from the germ-line inheritance of one or more mutant genes followed by additional somatic mutations. These two paths distinguish tumors that are characterized as **sporadic** and **hereditary**, respectively.

The role of epidemiology in human cancer biology

Epidemiology is the study of the distribution and determinants of disease frequency within a population. One of the earliest and most significant observations about human cancers is the striking relationship of most with age; the incidence increases at roughly the 3rd to 7th power of elapsed time. This observation has been interpreted to indicate that three to seven mutations are necessary before a cancer will form. Given the clonal origin of most solid neoplasms, these genetic mutations or 'hits' are thought to be sequential alterations of growth regulatory genes in a single cell and its progeny.

Epidemiologic associations have also identified environmental factors that increase the probability of a tumor developing. Examples of environmental factors are asbestos and estrogen; prolonged exposure to each dramatically increases the risk of lung and uterine cancers, respectively. Similarly, there are geographical clusters of specific cancers in regions of the world that share common dietary habits and other practices. These environmental factors probably abet the carcinogenic process by stimulating cell growth or turnover, thereby statistically increasing the rate of mutagenesis in actively dividing cells. Finally, epidemiologic studies identify subgroups of patients who may share a genetic predisposition to cancer such as the Ashkenazim.

Molecular biology of human cancers

Modern molecular biologic techniques have identified a number of common genes that are altered in neoplastic tissue. All the mutations identified to date occur in genes that are involved in some way in the regulation of normal cell proliferation. These genes fall into two major families: **oncogenes** and **tumor suppressor genes**. Oncogenes code for proteins whose function is to promote proliferation, and tumor suppressor genes for proteins that inhibit cell proliferation. Both mutational activation of proto-oncogenes to oncogenes and mutational inactivation of tumor suppressor genes *must* occur for a neoplasm to develop. Oncogene products are thus stimulatory to the tumor phenotype, and tumor suppressor gene products, inhibitory.

Proto-oncogenes, from which oncogenes form, are part of the normal genome. The function of proto-oncogenes is to drive cell proliferation at the appropriate time and place. An oncogene develops when a gain-of-function mutation occurs in a proto-oncogene. An oncogene, once activated, functions in a dominant fashion in the cell; this means that cell proliferation is stimulated when only one allele is affected. This class of genes was discovered through studies of retroviral tumorigenesis. Some retroviruses cause tumors by inserting viral genes that constitutively stimulate proto-oncogenes into vertebrate host cells, thereby inducing the tumor phenotype. There are two commonly observed mechanisms for mutational activation of human proto-oncogenes in solid tumors. The first is **gene amplification**, which typically results in overexpression of an otherwise normal protein. The second is **point mutation**, which leads to constitutive activation of a mutant form of the protein product.

Examples of commonly found human oncogenes are *ERBB2* (also known as *c-erbB2*/neu or *HER*-2/neu), *c-RAS*, *c-myc*, and *bcl*-2. *ERBB2* encodes for a transmembrane protein, p185, which shares considerable structural homology with the epidermal growth factor receptor (EGFR). Ligands such as EGF and transforming growth factor (TGF) bind to the extracellular domain of p185 and activate an intracellular tyrosine kinase signal transduction pathway. ***ERBB2* mutations affect cell proliferation.** The *c-ras* family of genes contains three members, *H-ras*, *K-ras* and *N-ras*. This oncogene family encodes for GTP binding proteins. The gene product of *K-ras*, $p21^{RAS}$, is a protein with GTPase activity tied to the adenylate cyclase signal transduction pathways. **$p21^{RAS}$ regulates progression of cells through the cell cycle.** *c-myc* codes for a leucine zipper type transcription factor. *bcl*-2 blocks a final common pathway leading to apoptosis.

Tumor suppressor genes normally encode for proteins whose function is to inhibit cell proliferation. Tumor suppressor genes are inactivated by loss-of-function mutations. In contrast to oncogenes, tumor suppressor genes act recessively at the cellular level; that is, both alleles must be inactivated for the tumor phenotype to be expressed. Point mutations, frameshift microdeletions or insertions, large deletions and translocations have all been identified in inactivated tumor suppressor genes. With only one known exception, hereditary cancer syndromes involve germ-line mutations in one tumor suppressor allele. This inherited mutation is revealed when the wild-type allele is inactivated by a second 'hit'. Most often, the second 'hit' is actual loss of the wild-type allele through mitotic non-disjunction, recombination error or deletion. This so-called **loss of heterozygosity (LOH)** is the hallmark of tumor suppressor gene inactivation.

Examples of tumor suppressor genes include *TP53*, *RB*, *WT1*, *NF1*, *APC*, *BRCA1* and *BRCA2*. ***TP53* is a cell checkpoint gene** located on chromosome 17p and is the best characterized tumor suppressor gene. p53, the gene product of *TP53*, is a multifunctional protein that is involved in transcription regulation, genomic stabilization, inhibition of cell cycle progression and apoptosis. Maintenance of wild-type p53 seems to be associated with sensitivity to chemotherapy; DNA damage done by the chemotherapy leads to activation of p53 and apoptosis of the damaged cells. *RB*, located on chromosome 13q, is associated with retinoblastoma susceptibility. *WT1* (chromosome 11p) is the Wilms' tumor gene and *DCC* (chromosome 18q) is the colon cancer gene. *NF1* (chromosome 17q) is associated with neurofibromatosis type 1. *APC* (chromosome 5q) is the gene involved in familial adenomatous polyposis coli. ***BRCA1* and *BRCA2* are the two inherited breast-cancer susceptibility genes.** *BRCA1* is located on chromosome 17q and, in addition to breast cancer, is associated with increased risk for ovarian and prostate cancers. *BRCA1* encodes for a protein that acts in conjunction with the hRAD51 systems to both repair double-stranded DNA breaks and regulate DNA transcription. *BRCA2* is located on chromosome 13q and inherited mutations in this locus confer risk largely for breast cancer. ***BRCA2*, like *BRCA1*, interacts with the hRAD51 system and confers genomic stability on cells.**

The discovery of the breast cancer susceptibility genes, *BRCA1* and *BRCA2*, led to a refinement of the original theory of inherited cancer syndromes. Initially, most of the inherited cancer susceptibility genes were thought to control cell proliferation directly, thereby acting in a 'gatekeeping' role. Subsequent to identification of *BRCA1* and *BRCA2* and investigations into the role of these two tumor suppressor genes, it became clear that genes that maintain the integrity of the genome, acting in a 'caretaking' role, may be even more frequent causes of inherited predispositions to cancer than gatekeepers. Gatekeeper genes directly affect the growth of tumors by inhibiting cell growth or promoting cell death. They are specific for cell types and inactivation of a given gatekeeper gene leads to a tissue-specific cancer. Examples of gatekeeper genes include *RB*, the retinoblastoma gene, and *APC*, the adenomatous polyposis coli gene, in which mutations lead to tumors of the retina and colon, respectively. People who have inherited one of these genes need only to have a mutation arise in the remaining wild-type allele and neoplasia will ensue. Because the probability of acquiring a single somatic mutation is exponentially greater than the probability of acquiring two such mutations randomly, people inheriting a mutant gatekeeper gene are at greater than a thousand-fold risk of developing these specific tumors than in the general population.

In contrast, inactivation of a caretaker gene like *BRCA1* or *BRCA2* does not promote tumor initiation directly. Instead inactivation of caretaker genes increases the statistical chance that other sporadic mutations will go undetected and uncorrected. People who inherit a caretaker gene mutation will not develop a tumor unless a mutation develops in the other caretaker gene, followed by mutations in both alleles of a gatekeeper gene. Because three additional mutations are necessary for tumorigenesis, people inheriting genes like *BRCA1* and *BRCA2* are only at 5–50 times the population risk for cancer. Other known caretaker genes include the mismatch-repair genes that cause hereditary non-polyposis colorectal cancer and the nucleotide-excision-repair genes that are responsible for xeroderma pigmentosum.

Genotype to phenotype models of cancer

Studies on tumor development have been conducted in both animal models and in humans. In animal models, the tumorigenic process is typically analysed in tumors deliberately induced by mutagenic agents, viruses or transgenes. From these animal experiments, we have learned that oncogenes such as c-*myc*, when transferred to a germ line under the control of a cell-specific promotor, will result in tumors of that cell progeny. However, even though all the cells contain the oncogene, only a few actually become neoplastic. This suggests that the presence of an oncogene alone is insufficient for neoplasia even if the gene is expressed at constitutively high levels for the lifetime of the animal. While doubly transgenic mice with two cell-specific oncogenes will develop tumors earlier and more frequently than single transgenic breeds, the proportion of neoplastic cells remains relatively small.

Studies in humans have shed light on why this occurs. In humans, the neoplastic process has been analysed through molecular characterization of the mutations occuring in sporadic tumors resected from patients. It is from the human data that the importance of tumor suppressor genes was identified. Oncogenes that inactivate tumor suppressor genes are particularly good at initiating tumorigenesis. One of the best examples of effective oncogene activity is the viral genes, *E6* and *E7*, of the human papilloma virus (Chapter 42.3). *E6* and *E7* appear to inactivate the products of two tumor suppressor genes, *p53* and *RB*, and initiate the neoplastic process in cervical cells. Inactivation of *p53* and *RB* by *E6* and *E7* are insufficient, however, to fully transform cells to the fully malignant state. Further unidentified hits are necessary.

Thus, the experimental data support the epidemiologic inference that multiple hits are necessary to transform even a germ-line genetic abnormality into a malignancy. The presence or absence of a precursor lesion in individual tumors has shaped how much we know about the sequence of events necessary for a specific cancer type to arise. Colorectal tumors, which progress through well defined morphological states during their development, are the first well characterized. A model for colorectal cancer is presented in part (a) of the figure below. Part (b) is an alternative model that fits the behavior of several other cancers, notably prostate. It better fits the non-linear molecular pathways that describe the abrupt changes seen in this tumor. The 'big bang' appears likely to be mutations in DNA repair genes (caretakers) that lead to exponential increases in risk for other mutations.

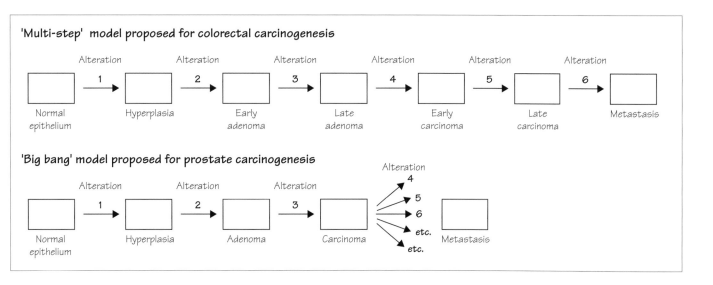

36 Breast cancer

Increasing odds: risk for women 20 years of age of developing breast cancer.

By age of	Number diagnosed with cancer
25	1 in 19 608
30	1 in 2525
35	1 in 622
40	1 in 217
45	1 in 93
50	1 in 50
55	1 in 33
60	1 in 24
65	1 in 17
70	1 in 14
75	1 in 11
80	1 in 10
85	1 in 9
Lifetime	1 in 8

Overview

Breast cancer is the most common malignancy in women and the second most frequent cause of cancer deaths in the United States. In addition to being predominantly a disease of women (99% of breast cancers occur in women), it is also a disease of aging. Although the lifetime risk of developing breast cancer for all women in the United States is 12%, this risk is largely concentrated in the perimenopausal and postmenopausal years. The effect of aging on breast cancer risk is not widely known among the public; older women tend to underestimate their risk and many women under 50 years of age grossly overestimate their risk. Consequently, these two groups of women misjudge the benefits of breast cancer screening programs.

Breast cancer may arise anywhere in the mammary gland. Tumors are typically classified by whether the cells of origin are lobular or ductal. Ductal carcinomas, which account for 85% of breast cancers, are either non-invasive (intraductal) or infiltrating. Intraductal carcinoma, also called ductal carcinoma *in situ* (DCIS), is defined histologically as carcinoma confined by the basement membrane of the duct. DCIS is considered a precursor lesion to invasive carcinoma as at least 33% of lesions will progress to invasive cancer in 5 years.

Once the basement membrane of the duct is breached, an infiltrating carcinoma has developed. The most common type of invasive carcinoma is ductal carcinoma (no special type), accounting for 79% of invasive carcinomas. The next most common type is lobular carcinoma, which arises from the terminal ductules of the alveoli and comprises 10% of invasive breast cancer. Less common types of infiltrating carcinomas include medullary and mucinous (colloid) carcinomas and Paget disease. Paget disease results when eczematous changes develop in the nipple and areola overlying an infiltrating ductal carcinoma in a main lactiferous duct. These skin changes are often the first sign of disease although the cancer may have been present for some time.

Breast cancer metastasizes first to the regional axillary lymph nodes. The most frequent distant metastatic sites are bone, liver, lung, pleura and brain. Patients with histologically negative axillary nodes have a much higher likelihood of survival than do patients with positive nodes. The ultimate prognosis is dependent on the size of the tumor, the number of involved nodes and the presence of lymphovascular invasion (LVI).

Treatment of invasive breast cancer is dependent on its stage and is typically multimodality. Surgical options include a modified radical mastectomy or lumpectomy with local irradiation, both with ipsilateral axillary node dissection. Antineoplastic chemotherapy is used more often in women who have positive nodes or negative nodes with a high risk of recurrence secondary to tumor size or LVI. Tamoxifen, which has both estrogenic and antiestrogenic properties, is the most widely used endocrine therapy for breast cancer. It is important to know the estrogen and progesterone receptor status of the tumor before considering endocrine therapy. The majority of receptor-positive tumors will respond to the antiestrogen, tamoxifen.

Treatment of DCIS is controversial and includes mastectomy or wide local excision which is often accompanied by irradiation. Recurrence

Determinants of breast cancer risk.

Factor	Relative risk
Family history of breast cancer	
First-degree relative	1.8
Premenopausal first-degree relative	3.0
Postmenopausal first-degree relative	1.5
Premenopausal first-degree relative (bilateral breast cancer)	9.0
Postmenopausal first-degree relative (bilateral breast cancer)	4.0–5.4
Menstrual history	
Menarche before age 12	1.7–3.4
Menarche after age 17	0.3
Menopause before age 45	0.5–0.7
Menopause from age 45 to 54	1.0
Menopause after age 55	1.5
Menopause after age 55 with more than 40 menstrual years	2.5–5.0
Oophorectomy before age 35	0.4
Anovulatory menstrual cycles	2.0–4.0
Pregnancy history	
Term pregnancy before age 20	0.4
First term pregnancy at age 20–34	1.0
First term pregnancy after age 35	1.5–4.0
Nulliparous patient	1.3–4.0
Histologic risk factors	
Atypical ductal hyperplasia	1.3–4.5
Atypical lobular hyperplasia	4.0
Lobular carcinoma *in situ*	5.4–12.0
Other	
Affluent vs. poor	2.0
Jewish vs. non-Jewish	2.0
Western hemisphere	1.5
Cold climate	1.5
Obesity + hypertension + diabetes	3.0
Moderate alcohol intake	1.3

rates following excision plus radiation are approximately 10%, half of which are invasive.

Epidemiology of breast cancer

The epidemiology of breast cancer in women suggests that it is an endocrine disorder related to prolonged exposure to ovarian hormones. Ovarian hormones have been shown to increase the mitotic activity of mammary cells in culture. In addition to the factors listed in the table opposite, hormonal treatment in the form of postmenopausal hormone replacement therapy may contribute to a higher lifetime risk of breast cancer.

There are also large ethnic and geographical differences in the prevalence of breast cancer throughout the world. Compared to American women, Asian women born and raised in Asia have one-fifth the risk of developing breast cancer. The risk rises toward the American level if Asians live in the United States for two or more generations, suggesting an environmental or lifestyle influence on the disease. Within the United States, the north-east has both the highest breast cancer and mortality rates. It has been suggested that the high incidence is due to a larger proportion of women in the region who delay their child-bearing. The association of alcohol intake and higher income with increased breast cancer risk supports an environmental influence on its development.

Familial breast cancer

About 10% of breast cancer is familial. The clustering of breast cancers with ovarian cancers in many familial cases led to the discovery of two genes, *BRCA1* and *BRCA2*, in which germ-line mutations predispose to formation of specific cancers. Current evidence indicates that 75% of inherited cases of breast cancer are the results of mutations involving *BRCA1* and *BRCA2*. Both *BRCA1* and *BRCA2* are tumor suppressor genes and thus both alleles must be abnormal before tumorigenesis will occur. The ethnic and geographic distributions of *BRCA1* and *BRCA2* are discussed in Chapter 39.

Molecular biology of sporadic (non-familial) breast cancer

Molecular studies have identified a number of abnormal loci that occur with high frequency in breast cancer specimens but not in normal breast tissue. The most commonly encountered abnormalities involve the oncogenes, *ERBB2* and c-*myc*, the tumor suppressor gene *TP53*, and telomerase. Both oncogenes are amplified or overexpressed in about 30% of breast cancers whereas telomerase activity is elevated in 80–90%. Breast tissue with *ERBB2* abnormalities appears to be resistant to the effects of the antiestrogen tamoxifen but more chemosensitive. *TP53* abnormalities interfere with normal apoptosis, thereby making affected tumors more resistant to chemotherapy and radiation therapy.

Breast cancer, like most malignancies, probably results from the effects of environmental triggers in a genetically susceptible tissue. Genetic susceptibility may result from germline mutations like *BRCA1* and *BRCA2* or from abnormalities arising during intrauterine or pubertal differentiation. Environmental influences such as prolonged ovarian hormone exposure may increase mitogenesis in the breast, predisposing mammary ductal epithelium to further genomic damage and transformation from atypical benign cells to a malignancy. Other environmental influences such as pregnancy may enhance differentiation and reduce the risk of an abnormal response to normal growth factors.

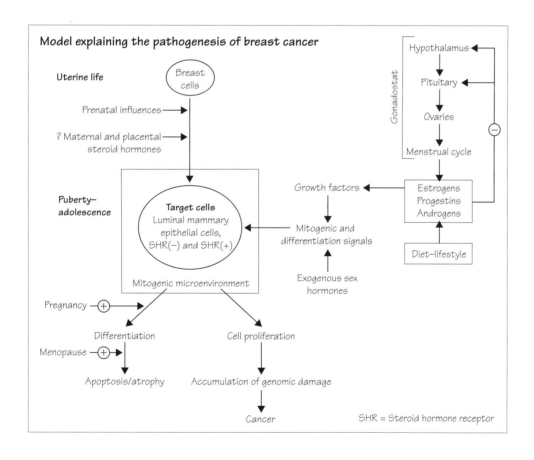

Hypothetical scheme of human testicular germ cell tumor development						
Type of germ cells / DNA characteristics	Primordial germ cells	Spermatogonia	Binucleated dysplastic germ cells	Atypical germ cells	Seminoma cells	Cells of embryonal carcinoma
Ploidy	Euploid	Euploid	Euploid/ Aneuploid	Aneuploid	Aneuploid	Aneuploid
Number of chromosome 1 in interphase nuclei	?	2	?	2, 3, 4	2, 3, (4)	2, 3
Modal chromosome number	46, XY	46, XY	?	70–80, XY	70–80, XY	55–65, XY

Evolution of germ cell tumors

Activation 1   Activation 2

Overview

Testicular cancer is the most common malignancy in men in the 20–40-year age group. The incidence of the most prevalent type of testicular cancer, the germ-cell tumors (GCTs), has risen over the past two decades, as has the most prevalent risk factor for GCT, an undescended testis (cryptorchidism). This suggests that the number of men afflicted with testicular cancer will continue to rise for the foreseeable future.

Unlike ovarian tumors, which are most likely to arise from the epithelium covering the gland, 90% of primary testicular tumors arise from intratubular germ cells. Histologically, there are six distinct types of GCT, five of which occur in young men and one which is seen exclusively in older men. The five subtypes seen in young men include **seminoma**, **choriocarcinoma**, **yolk sac carcinoma** (endodermal sinus tumor), **embryonal carcinoma** and **teratomas**, both benign and malignant. Spermatocytic seminomas typically are seen in men over 50 years of age and are quite rare by comparison to the other GCTs. The distinction between the GCT of young and old men is important not only because of the histopathologic differences, but because the germ cells of origin appear to be at different stages of maturation. Hence the tumors have very different neoplastic behaviors.

GCTs of young men all appear to arise from spermatogonial cells. The five tumors that develop from this single precursor cell type are quite heterogeneous and several exhibit embryonal-like differentiation. As such, these tumors provide a unique opportunity for the analysis of the genetic basis of malignant transformation and differentiation of a stem cell system. Prognosis and treatment depends upon whether GCTs are pure seminomas (SGCTs) or mixed cell (non-seminomas; NSGCTs). Seminomas have a distinct and homogeneous germ-cell

morphology. Non-seminomas present features of the embryonal cells and can mimic the histogenesis of the very early embryo. Embryonal carcinoma is the most primitive, or pluripotent of the NSGCTs. It can progress along extraembryonic lines as choriocarcinoma or yolk sac carcinoma or along embryonic lines as a teratoma. Individual tumors can contain a mixture of any of the histologic types.

About 80% of GCTs secrete tumor markers which can be detected in the serum of patients. Tumors with yolk sac components typically secrete alfafetoprotein (AFP), an embryonic protein produced normally during development by the yolk sac and subsequently by the fetal liver. Other NSGCTs can secrete AFP but seminomas do not. Human chorionic gonadotropin (hCG) is typically secreted by choriocarcinomas; however, small amounts of hCG production have been found in SGCTs as well as NSGCTs. The distribution of these two markers by specific cell types suggests that they arise from precursors at different levels of differentiation. AFP is a very primitive marker of embryonal differentiation whereas hCG represents trophoblastic differentiation. A third marker, placental-like alkaline phosphatase (PLAP), is found in carcinoma *in situ* (CIS) and about 50% of seminomas. Clinical paradigms using serum levels of AFP and hCG, have been developed to assist in the diagnosis and staging of GCT.

Most GCTs are diagnosed at an early tumor stage when the tumor is confined to the testis. Serum screening, physical exam and testicular ultrasounds are useful in identifying early tumors in patients at high risk for GCT such as formerly cryptorchid men and intersex individuals who will keep their gonads. Men who present with solid testicular masses are usually treated by radical orchidectomy (removal of the testis). When GCT metastasizes, it typically spreads to the unilateral para-aortic nodes and less commonly to the contralateral chain. Continuous spread throughout the lymphatic system occurs with positive nodes appearing in the posterior mediastinum and supraclavicular chain. Supradiaphragmatic spread occurs via the thoracic duct. Pulmonary and brain metastases are generally found only in tumors with trophoblast components.

GCT, like gestational trophoblast disease in women (Chapter 34.6), has a very high cure rate such that virtually all patients with early stage disease can expect to be cured. Initial treatment of stage I disease is typically removal of the affected testes followed by either abdominopelvic lymph node dissection, a short course of adjuvant chemotherapy or close surveillance. Even metastatic disease is amenable to chemotherapy with cure rates in excess of 90%.

Leydig cell tumors are a very rare form of testicular cancer (1–3%) and are associated with isosexual precocious puberty (Chapter 26). **Gonadal stromal tumors** (sex cord-stromal tumors), which include both Leydig–Sertoli cell and granulosa-theca cell tumors, are extraordinarily rare in boys and men and are associated with feminization.

Epidemiology of GCT

The single largest risk factor for GCT is cryptorchidism (Chapter 24). It is estimated that 2–3% of cryptorchid men will develop GCT, a relative risk five to 10 times that of the general population. GCT disproportionately affects white men of European descent and is uncommon in African and Asian men, independent of where they live. Familial cases are also common; the pedigrees suggest that a single dominant gene with low penetrance is involved in these cases.

The strong developmental association of cryptorchidism and hormonal abnormalities suggests that fetal or neonatal endocrine imbalances may be involved in the initiation of GCT. One clue to the possible nature of the imbalance is the higher incidence of testicular cancer, cryptorchidism and hypospadias seen among the sons of women who were treated with the synthetic estrogen diethylstilbestrol (DES) between 1945 and 1971. This DES effect has led to the hypothesis that overexposure to estrogens in fetal development may provide 'activation 1' leading to CIS formation with its aneuploidy and p12 abnormalities. These increased levels of maternal estrogen can suppress the fetal pituitary production of follicle-stimulating hormone (FSH) through negative feedback. Less FSH leads to reduced Sertoli cell multiplication and lower levels of Müllerian-inhibiting substance (MIS). The increased estrogens may also impair Leydig cell function, thereby decreasing local androgen production and testicular descent. MIS has been implicated as necessary for both the normal descent of the testes and normal differentiation of fetal gonocytes into type A spermatogonia. Over the past 20 years, maternal estrogen ingestion in the form of phytestrogens (soya) and chemical pollutants with estrogenic activity has increased, as has the incidence of both cryptorchidism and GCT.

Exposure of the cryptorchid testes to high temperatures may also play a role in the development of GCT, as the maturation of gonocytes to type A spermatogonia is significantly inhibited in abdominal testes. This does not fully explain the role of cryptorchidism, however, as maldescended testes that have been restored to the scrotum in infancy or childhood still retain an increased lifetime risk of GCT as does the contralateral testis in cases of unilateral cryptorchidism.

Molecular biology of GCT

Cytogenetic studies on GCTs in all the histological subsets demonstrate sex chromosome constitutions of XY, confirming the origin of GCT in germ cells prior to the first meiotic division. They also have aneuploid chromosome numbers, typically almost triploid. Almost all tumors have multiple copies of chromosome 12p, either as one or more copies of i(12p) or as tandemly duplicated segments of 12p on marker chromosomes. Deletions of 12q are frequent. These findings have led to the following model of tumorigenesis in GCT.

The precursor cell for GCT is the pachytene spermatocyte, which has a 4C DNA content from the final DNA replication in the premeiotic spermatogonial cell (Chapters 7 and 15). At this stage, the homologous autosomes are paired as bivalents and the sex chromosomes are aligned. These chromosomes will then undergo crossing-over and segregate as they progress to metaphase 1. The process of crossing-over requires activation of specific genes to repair the resulting open chromosomal ends. If, for any reason, the repair mechanism fails, the individual spermatocyte cannot progress any further and degenerates. A meiosis stage cell with a defective repair mechanism is rescued from death only by initiation of a new program for mitotic division. Such a proliferation is neoplastic. In the 4C spermatocyte, the aberrant chromatid exchange event that initiates the new cell cycle must involve a locus on p12, given that it is almost uniformly abnormal in GCT. Either the locus is inverted as i(p12) or tandem duplication occurs providing the necessary extra copy number and presumably increased gene product to rescue the cell from death. Initiation of another round of DNA replication in the 4C cell will lead to a tetraploid cell with an i(p12) or amplified p12. Because the initial repair defect remains, the cell is genetically unstable and liable to undergo other chromosomal changes such as non-disjunction, mutation and microdeletion. Aberrations in the locus *PT53*, which are common in a number of other neoplastic processes, do not appear to play a role in GCT. Actually, the above model presumes wild-type (normal) p53, which is necessary to regulate apoptosis, or programmed cell death, in cells with DNA damage. In such cells, p53 can initiate cell cycle arrest, enabling repair of DNA lesions before restoration of the normal cell cycle or, if DNA damage is excessive, p53 can initiate apoptosis. Intact p53 may explain, in part, why GCT is exquisitely sensitive to chemotherapy (Chapter 35).

It is not clear whether all GCTs derive clonally from a single cell that has undergone malignant transformation or whether tumorigenesis can be multifocal. An alternate, but related, hypothesis to the one above is that a subset of gonocytes undergo 'activation 1' in which they become bi- or multinucleated spermatogonia. Subsequently, nuclear fusion

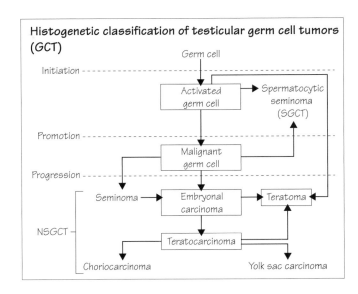

Histogenetic classification of testicular germ cell tumors (GCT)

occurs in some of these abnormal spermatogonia and they become tetraploid cells. These aneuploid cells then receive a 'second hit' or 'activation 2' and lose specific genes or chromosomes that are important for tumor suppression. The clonality or multifocality of a given tumor might then depend on the specific activating factors.

Regardless of how these cells undergo malignant transformation, it is clear that tumorigenesis can occur in infancy or even prenatally, perhaps as early as during testicular differentiation. Testicular CIS, a polyploid non-invasive precursor to GCT that shares the aneuploidy and 12p amplifications of GCT, has been found in both fetal and neonatal testes. Given that the peak incidence of frankly invasive carcinoma occurs two to three decades after precursor lesions may be found, GCT appears to have a very long latency. The long latency lends support to the second hit or activation theory in the development of GCT. In addition, early hormonal imbalances, particularly androgen exposure at puberty, may also play a role in the development of GCT, perhaps in the 'activation 2' step.

In contrast to GCT in young men, the spermatocytic seminomas seen in older men are more indolent and slow growing. This less aggressive behavior may occur because spermatocytic seminomas appear to arise from mature spermatogonia and not spermatogonial stem cells. A molecular basis for the different biological behavior may lie in the imprinting that occurs between the second meiotic division of germ cells and the mature spermatocyte. Molecular genetic studies have demonstrated the importance of converting the biparental diploid genotype of the gonadal stem cell into not only a haploid cell, but also one that is totally uniparental. This imprinting is thought to occur sometime during spermatocyte maturation but after the second meiotic division that halves the chromosome number. The biparental imprinting of the early meiotic spermatogonia may preserve the pluripotentiality of the transformed cells, thereby permitting development into either embryonal or trophoblastic components in addition to the seminomas. Parental imprinting of the mature spermatogonium would lead to the less aggressive spermatocytic seminomas.

Diseases of the prostate

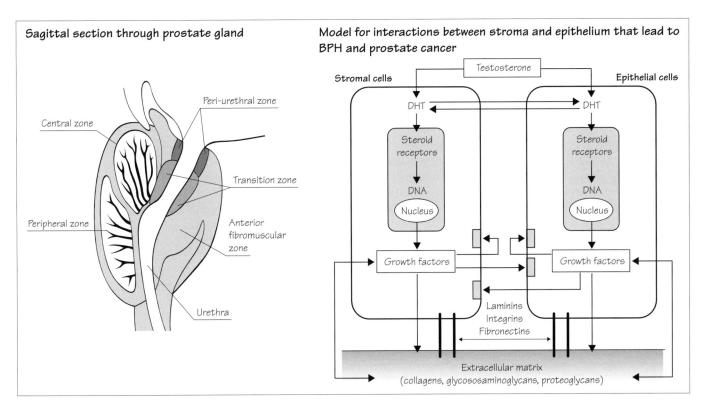

Sagittal section through prostate gland

Central zone

Peri-urethral zone

Transition zone

Peripheral zone

Anterior fibromuscular zone

Urethra

Model for interactions between stroma and epithelium that lead to BPH and prostate cancer

Testosterone

Stromal cells

Epithelial cells

DHT

DHT

Steroid receptors

Steroid receptors

DNA

DNA

Nucleus

Nucleus

Growth factors

Growth factors

Laminins
Integrins
Fibronectins

Extracellular matrix
(collagens, glycososaminoglycans, proteoglycans)

1 BENIGN PROSTATIC HYPERTROPHY

Overview

The prostate is the organ of the body most frequently afflicted by disease in males over 50 years of age. The single most common pathologic process is benign prostatic hypertrophy (BPH). At least 70% of 70-year-old men develop BPH and 40% of them suffer from some symptom of bladder outflow obstruction.

Epidemiology and symptoms

The single clearly documented risk factor for BPH is age. Data suggesting that black race puts men at increased risk appears to be poorly controlled for socioeconomic status and access to health care.

BPH will cause urethral obstruction severe enough to warrant medical intervention in about 30% of elderly men. There is not a good correlation between the size of the prostate and either the presence or severity of outflow obstruction. In addition to physical obstruction of the urethra, BPH can also produce irritative symptoms. These include frequency and urgency of micturition, urge incontinence and nocturia. It is felt by some that the irritative symptoms are the result of partial denervation of the tissue that occurs with fibromuscular hypertrophy.

BPH is characterized by a gradual increase in both the glandular and fibromuscular tissue in the periurethral and transition zones of the prostate. The periurethral and transition zones surround the urethra at its origin from the bladder and midsegment, respectively. Nodular hyperplasia, the characteristic change of BPH, is not simply an increase

in the cell population of the gland, but changes in the architecture of the ducts and acini. In periurethral-zone BPH, the nodular hyperplasia consists of a mixture of glandular and fibromuscular elements often with fibromuscular proliferation to the exclusion of the epithelium. BPH occurring in the transition zone is characterized by large amounts of glandular tissue that arises by budding and branching of pre-existing ducts. This type of hyperplastic proliferation is a highly unusual finding in any other tissue, whether normal or diseased, in the adult human. It is felt that this anomalous behavior results from a reversion of the tissue to its embryonic behavior.

Pathogenesis

Different embryologic origins of tissues within the prostate may explain why **BPH occurs within the transition and central zones** while prostatic adenocarcinoma occurs within the peripheral zone. The transition and central zones appear to be of Wolffian duct derivation while the peripheral zone arises from the urogenital sinus (Chapter 5.3).

A normally functioning testis is a prerequisite for developing BPH, as is the presence of functional 5α-reductase. Prostate development is unique among the internal genitalia in that it requires dihydrotestosterone (DHT) both embryologically and for maintenance. Testosterone acts as a prohormone that is converted to the more potent prostatic androgen DHT by 5α-reductase in the stromal cells of the gland. DHT is more potent than testosterone because of the higher affinity of the prostatic nuclear androgen receptor for DHT. Individuals lacking 5α-reductase have a vestigial prostate and never develop BPH or prostate cancer.

Differentiation and growth of prostatic epithelium is dependent on androgen-sensitive factors made in the underlying stroma (embryologic mesenchyme). Candidate growth factors, which increase mitosis in prostatic epithelial cells *in vitro*, include epidermal growth factor (EGF), insulin-like growth factors (IGFs) and basic fibroblast growth factor (bFGF). Transforming growth factor β_2 (TGF-β_2) decreases the mitotic activity. Expression of bFGF is increased in BPH.

Men with BPH have increased 5α-reductase activity and possibly an increase in prostate androgen receptors making the 'aging' prostate more susceptible to androgen stimulation. Gene expression for the growth factors bFGF and TGF-β_2 is increased in BPH. There may be a protective role for estrogens in BPH. Estradiol production slowly increases in older men as the testes become less responsive to luteinizing hormone (LH) and more LH is required to maintain androgen production. Estrogen production is disproportionately stimulated by high LH and, in turn, the estrogen increases hepatic sex hormone-binding globulin (SHBG) synthesis. More SHBG reduces the concentration of free testosterone in the circulation, thereby also reducing the amount available to be converted to DHT in the prostatic stroma.

Treatment of BPH

Treatment of BPH traditionally has been surgical resection via transurethral prostatectomy (TURP). TURP is the second most common operation performed in men over the age of 65 years. Medical treatment with α-adrenergic agents such as prazosin, ketanserin or terazosin will improve obstructive voiding symptoms and urine flow; these medications are effective because of the large proportion of smooth muscle containing adrenergic receptors in BPH. Effective α-adrenergic agents have significant side-effects. The specific dependence of the pro-static epithelium on DHT has led to the development of the 5α-reductase inhibitor, finasteride, which shrinks the prostate and improves symptoms with fewer side-effects. Naturally occurring phytoestrogens are purported to have an effect but have not been tested in controlled trials.

2 PROSTATE CANCER

Overview

Prostate cancer (PCa) is the most common non-cutaneous malignancy in the United States and Europe and it is likely to grow in frequency as the population ages. Autopsy series have consistently found incidental PCa in 15–45% of older men.

Epidemiology

Risk factors for PCa include age, race, positive family history, dietary fat intake, circulating hormone levels and possibly vasectomy. African-American men who consume a high fat diet are at highest risk for PCa and Asian men living in the Far East on a low fat diet carry the lowest risk. Changes in geography or eating habits have a profound modifying effect on the background racial difference. Plasma androgen concentrations at the high end of normal increase the risk of PCa as do sex hormone-binding globulin (SHBG) or estrogen concentrations at the lower end of the normal range. Obstruction of the vas deferens by vasectomy causes death of the seminiferous epithelium and Sertoli cells, leading to Leydig cell hyperplasia and increased local testosterone concentrations in the testicular veins.

As with most malignancies, PCa probably occurs as a result of environmental promoters in a genetically susceptible tissue. For PCa, age and family history are predisposing factors whereas androgen is the promoter. The impact of race and geography may not be in susceptibility because the incidence of microscopic PCa appears independent of both, in spite of markedly different incidence rates of clinically apparent disease. The progression of latent tumors to clinically evident tumors is a rate-limiting step which race appears to influence. Modest differences in androgen production among African-American, Asian and white men have been found and over a lifetime may explain the influence of race on PCa.

A positive family history, while it confers significant risk for an individual in that family, accounts for only a small number of the cases of PCa. The hereditary form is distinguished from the more common form by an earlier age of onset.

Pathogenesis

The most common form of PCa is adenocarcinoma of the glandular epithelium of the peripheral zone of the prostate gland. Adenocarcinoma of the prostate appears to be the end result of androgen activity upon a vulnerable substrate, that is, one that has acquired oncogenic potential. The first signs of an evolving neoplastic process are proliferation and anaplasia of the cells lining the ducts and glandular acini of the **peripheral zone**. This lesion is called **prostatic intraepithelial neoplasia (PIN)**. Disruption of the architecture of the basal epithelial cell layers is common in PIN.

Like most malignancies, the prognosis in PCa is determined by both the stage and grade of the tumor at detection. Disease localized to the prostate has about 80% survival at 5 years whereas the presence of distant metastases significantly lowers 5-year survival. PCa spreads locally to the hypogastric and presacral chains of lymph nodes and hematogenously to bone.

Prostate-specific antigen (PSA) is a protease that is secreted by the epithelium into prostatic secretions. Small amounts leak into the plasma across the prostatic acini. PSA determinations have been used as a screening tool for PCa in asymptomatic men with variable results. The cost effectiveness of PSA screening is still under debate.

At the cellular level, the interaction between prostatic stroma and epithelium appears to play an important role in the development of PCa. Different stromal growth factors are overexpressed in PCa when compared to BPH. Specifically, the stroma of PCa contains more IGF, EGF and TGF-β in contrast to overexpression of bFGF in BPH. DHT and testosterone both stimulate production of EGF and TGF-β by the prostate gland. The androgen dependence of these growth factors probably accounts for much of the hormonal dependence of the gland.

EGF receptor (EGFR) activity is overexpressed in PCa as a result of mutations in the *ERBB2* oncogene. Overexpression of *ERBB2* is also found in breast cancer. In both prostate and breast cancer, the EGFR shifts from the basal epithelial layer to the luminal epithelium as the disease progresses from hyperplasia to intraepithelial neoplasia to frank cancer. Families, in which PCa clusters, frequently carry mutations in the *BRCA1* or *BRCA2* tumor suppressor genes. Mutations in these genes are also associated with breast and ovarian cancers.

Several chromosomal loci have been identified as potential sites for tumor suppressor activity in PCa using loss of heterogeneity (LOH) assays. The commonly identified *TP53* tumor suppressor locus does not seem as important in PCa as it does in other tumors. Interestingly, in PCa that metastasizes after therapy, there is a gain in genetic material at a locus on the short arm of the X chromosome. The Xq site appears to contain the gene for the androgen receptor (AR) that becomes amplified after treatment with androgen withdrawal; that is, there is an increase in number of copies of the AR gene when androgen is removed from the environment. This acquired defect is thought to represent an adaptation that improves the ability of the cells to survive and grow under androgen-deficient conditions. The discovery of AR gene amplification in PCa after androgen withdrawal therapy has provided important insight into the molecular basis for the development of drug resistance by cancer cells.

Treatment

Treatment of PCa can be either surgery or irradiation for local disease, and irradiation combined with androgen ablation for more widespread disease. The choice of surgical extirpation or irradiation may be individualized based on age, operative risk and patient choice. Androgen withdrawal may be accomplished by orchidectomy; by treatment with a luteinizing hormone-releasing hormone (LHRH) agonist such as goserelin or leuprolide; or by treatment with one of the antiandrogens such as flutamide, bicalutamide or nilutamide. Chemotherapy has not been shown to be effective in treating PCa probably because of a slow doubling time for the tumor combined with technical difficulties in quantifying the extent of the tumor burden at the beginning and end of therapy.

39 Ovarian neoplasms

Overview

It is estimated that 5–10% of women in the United States will undergo a surgical procedure for a suspected ovarian neoplasm at some time during their lifetime. Fortunately, the overwhelming majority of ovarian masses are benign; the lifetime risk of developing ovarian cancer is about 2%. Age is the most important factor in determining risk of malignancy. During the reproductive years, adnexal masses are common and are usually functional cysts or benign neoplasms of the ovary or postinfectious changes in the Fallopian tubes. In both girls under the age of 20 and women over 50 years of age, a palpable ovarian mass is malignant about 10% of the time. Between 85% and 90% of all ovarian cancer occurs in postmenopausal women.

Benign neoplasms of the ovary

Benign, as well as malignant neoplasms, can develop from any cell type found in the ovary. Simple cysts arising from the ovulation site (functional) or corpus luteum are very common and can be distinguished from true neoplasms by their transitory nature. They will typically disappear within 6 weeks of discovery. Complex or solid masses are more likely to be truly neoplastic and require histological diagnosis. With few exceptions, benign neoplasms of the ovary are not premalignant lesions that progress to invasive cancer. Thus, careful screening and removal of benign and borderline tumors of the ovary over the last 20 years has not reduced the incidence of ovarian cancer.

Ovarian cancers

Ovarian cancers stand in stark contrast to those of the testes where 90% of the malignancies are germ-cell tumors that have early detection and high cure rates (Chapter 37). Ninety per cent of ovarian malignancies are epithelial cell cancers. When detected after widespread intraperitoneal dissemination, cure is almost impossible.

There are four distinct histological types of epithelial ovarian cancer: serous, mucinous, endometrioid and clear cell. Of the four, serous cancers account for almost half of all tumors. Mucinous and endometrioid cancers each occur in about 15% of cases. Clear cell cancers account for only 6% of the total.

Epithelial ovarian cancer typically spreads both locally and by intraperitoneal dissemination. Contiguous spread is to the Fallopian tube and uterus and dissemination occurs to the contralateral ovary and peritoneum. Implants may be found on the cul-de-sac, bowel, mesentery, omentum and diaphragm. Malignant ascites forms when diaphragmatic metastases block the lymphatic drainage of the peritoneal cavity. Patients are asymptomatic until either they develop symptoms related to a mass effect or the ascites causes abdominal bloating, dyspepsia or urinary frequency. The lack of early symptoms leads to late diagnosis and poor prognosis. Treatment for epithelial ovarian cancer is cytoreductive surgery and aggressive chemotherapy; only 15% of patients with advanced disease will survive because of eventual development of tumor resistance to chemotherapy. When disease is confined to the ovary, survival is dramatically improved to 50–90%.

About 15% of all epithelial ovarian cancers have histologic and biologic behaviors that are between clearly benign and frankly malignant

Histogenetic classification of ovarian neoplasms.

Neoplasms derived from coelomic epithelium
Serous tumor
Mucinous tumor
Endometrioid tumor
Mesonephroid (clear cell) tumor
Brenner tumor
Carcinosarcoma and mixed mesodermal tumor

Neoplasms derived from germ cells
Teratoma
  Mature teratoma
    Solid adult teratoma
    Dermoid cyst
    Struma ovarii
    Malignant neoplasms secondarily arising from mature cystic teratoma
  Immature teratoma (partially differentiated teratoma)
Dysgerminoma
Embryonal carcinoma
Endodermal sinus tumor
Choriocarcinoma
Gonadoblastoma

Neoplasms derived from specialized gonadal stroma
Granulosa-theca cell tumors
  Granulosa tumor
  Thecoma
Sertoli–Leydig tumors
  Arrhenoblastoma
  Sertoli tumor
Gynandroblastoma
Lipid cell tumors

Neoplasms derived from non-specific mesenchyme
Fibroma, hemangioma, leiomyoma, lipoma
Lymphoma
Sarcoma

Neoplasms metastatic to the ovary
Gastrointestinal tract (Krukenberg)
Breast
Endometrium
Lymphoma

---

neoplasms. These borderline tumors have a 95% 10-year survival but can recur as many as 20 years after excision. It is unclear whether or not some borderline ovarian cancers are precursors to frankly malignant tumors. Late recurrences are often identical to the primary tumor, but malignant transformation to high-grade epithelial ovarian cancer is also seen.

Familial ovarian cancer

There are three recognized cancer predisposition syndromes, which include ovarian cancer: familial ovarian cancer syndrome, hereditary breast/ovarian cancer syndrome and Lynch cancer family syndrome II (hereditary non-polyposis colorectal cancer syndrome; HNPCC). These syndromes account for less than 10% of the ovarian cancer diagnoses. Virtually all of the hereditary breast/ovarian cancers and site-specific ovarian cancer syndromes are caused by *BRCA1* or *BRCA2* mutations, the tumor suppressor genes originally identified with susceptibility to early onset breast cancer. Individuals with *BRCA1* mutations have a 20-fold increase in risk for developing both breast and ovarian cancers, whereas *BRCA2* carriers have a 5–10-fold increase in risk for ovarian cancers. The most common extracolonic malignancy in women with HNPCC is endometrial cancer, followed by ovarian cancer. Any one of three genes important in mismatch repair is mutated in this syndrome.

The estimated frequency of *BRCA1* mutations in the general population is 1/800, but is greater than 1/100 among Ashkenazi Jewish women. *BRCA2* mutations have a very similar carrier frequency as *BRCA1* among the Ashkenazim and occur with a frequency of 1/250 among Icelanders.

Epidemiology of epithelial ovarian cancer

Next to a strong family history, age is the single largest risk factor for epithelial ovarian cancer with the mean onset at age 59 years. Other risk factors for epithelial ovarian cancer are early menarche, regular periods, shorter menstrual cycle length, low parity and prolonged use of ovulation induction for treatment of infertility. High parity and use of oral contraceptives, both of which decrease the number of ovulations, reduce the risk of ovarian cancer. These epidemiologic data suggest that the number of ovulations over a lifetime is significant in the pathogenesis of the disease.

As with other prevalent epithelial cancers, epidemiologic evidence also strongly suggests that environmental factors play a role in the development of ovarian cancers. The highest rates of ovarian cancer are found in highly industrialized countries with Japan as the single notable exception. In Japan, rates of malignant neoplasms of the ovary are among the lowest in the world. The rates in Japanese immigrants in the United States approach those of Caucasian natives within two to three generations. These findings suggest that carcinogens within the immediate environment such as food or personal customs are responsible. Chemical carcinogens from the outside world can reach the pelvic peritoneum of women through the vagina and upper reproductive tract; in one study, more women with ovarian cancer had used talc as a dusting powder on their perineum or sanitary napkins than had matched controls. The association between talc and ovarian cancer is biologically plausible because talc is chemically related to asbestos and ovarian cancer is similar to the mesotheliomas that can develop with asbestos exposure of the lung.

Molecular biology of non-familial epithelial ovarian cancer

Biologic study of epithelial ovarian cancers has been hampered by their advanced stage at clinical presentation and by the lack of identifiable precursor lesions for the more common serous and mucinous adenocarcinomas. Some investigators believe that epithelial ovarian cancers arise in small inclusion cysts that develop when surface epithelial cells become entrapped in ovulatory defects. Another theory is that ovarian epithelium is coelomic mesothelium that is more prone to metaplasia than other epithelia. Both theories are consistent with the epidemiologic data suggesting that events that disrupt the integrity of the ovarian capsule predispose to tumorigenesis.

As with other malignancies, ovarian cancer probably develops after multiple genetic 'hits' cause a cell to display invasive, neoplastic behavior. One 'hit' typically involves activation of an oncogene and the second 'hit' is the loss of one or more genes with tumor suppressor activity. Recurrent disruption and repair of the ovarian capsular epithelium could lead to increased risk of activation of proto-oncogenes, as could environmental insults that disrupt the coelomic mesothelium. *BRCA1* and *BRCA2* are tumor suppressor genes and inheritance of one abnormal allele makes 'second hits' a high statistical probability.

Oncogenes that have been identified with high frequency in non-familial cases of epithelial ovarian cancer include *ERBB2*, whose cellular homolog is the epithelial growth factor (EGF) receptor gene, and c-*fms* whose cellular homolog is the macrophage colony-stimulating factor (M-CSF) receptor gene. The most commonly found tumor suppressor abnormalities involve p53, the product of a tumor suppressing cell checkpoint gene located on chromosome 17p. Fifty per cent of ovarian cancers overexpress p53, and allelic losses on chromosome 17p are found in up to 75% of ovarian cancers. Point mutations and loss of *PT53* are not found in benign or borderline ovarian tumors consistent with their lack of precursor status. Mucinous cancers of the ovary frequently show point mutations of the K-*ras* oncogene.

Endometrioid and clear cell cancers of the ovary, while rare, may be the exception to the rule that epithelial ovarian cancers do not have well defined premalignant lesions that progress to invasive cancer. Both cancer types have been found nested within areas of endometriosis on the ovary and common loss of heterozygosity (LOH) events are seen in the adjacent endometrial tissue and the cancer. There is about a 1% risk of malignant transformation of ovarian endometriosis.

Other ovarian malignancies

Germ-cell tumors (GCTs) account for only 10% of ovarian cancers and occur largely in girls and young women. Like GCTs in men, GCTs in women arise from immature germ cells and include five distinct histological types: **dysgerminoma**, **choriocarcinoma**, **yolk sac carcinoma** (endodermal sinus tumor), **embryonal carcinoma** and **teratomas**. The dysgerminoma is the female equivalent of the seminoma. Because GCTs of the ovary are not detected early in their development as are GCTs of the testes, far less is known about GCT tumorigenesis in the female than in the male (Chapter 37).

Benign ovarian teratomas are also known as **dermoids** and represent a unique subclass of the female germ-cell tumors because they arise from more mature germ cells than the other GCTs. Grossly, dermoids contain hair, bone, cartilage and a large amount of greasy fluid that rapidly becomes sebaceous at room temperature. Histologically, one sees many of the cell types normally seen in fetuses, all in disarray. Like other GCTs, the molecular event(s) that lead to activation of the germ cells can occur *in utero* and indeed, dermoid tumors have been detected in the fetus and newborn. They arise by 'parthenogenetic' activation of premeiotic oocytes. Modern molecular techniques have demonstrated that all of the chromosomes are maternally imprinted. The contribution of dermoid cysts to our understanding of early embryonic development is discussed in Chapter 15.

Stromal cell tumors are the rarest of ovarian malignancies and account for only 5% of the total. These tumors may contain granulosa, theca, Leydig or Sertoli cells. The tumors usually make large amounts of steroid hormones; granulosa or theca cell tumors make estrogens and Leydig or Sertoli cell tumors make androgens. Stromal cell tumors are not age dependent and can be associated with virilization.

40 Endometrial cancer

Overview

Carcinoma of the uterine endometrium is the most common pelvic malignancy in women. The United States and Canada have the highest incidence rates in the world, whereas developing countries and Japan have incidence rates four to five times lower. Epidemiologic data indicate that there are two forms of endometrial cancer; one which is directly related to estrogen exposure and is most common in the United States, and another which is unrelated to estrogen and occurs throughout the world. Type I tumors, which are estrogen related, occur in relatively younger perimenopausal women and are associated with a good prognosis. Type II tumors, which are not estrogen related, occur in older postmenopausal women without a history of estrogen exposure and are associated with a poorer prognosis. In addition to the presence or absence of specific clinical characteristics, two different profiles of molecular genetic alterations appear to be present in type I and type II endometrial carcinomas. Most importantly for the clinician, the type I lesions are potentially preventable through recognition of patient risk, diagnosis of the precursor lesion (atypical endometrial hyperplasia) and proper treatment.

Endometrioid adenocarcinoma is by far the most common histological subtype of endometrial cancer. Histological grade of endometrioid adenocarcinoma (well, moderately or poorly differentiated) is an important prognostic indicator independent of tumor stage. The other, less common, subtypes reflect the wide potential for differentiation of the Müllerian tract. Other subtypes include mucinous, serous and clear cell adenocarcinoma, squamous carcinoma and a variety of rare mixed and undifferentiated tumors. Prognosis of the subtypes other than endometrioid adenocarcinoma is more dependent on the type of originating cell than on the histological grade of the neoplasia.

Endometrioid adenocarcinoma first invades the stroma of the tissue by destroying the glandular basement membrane. It typically then invades the myometrium and cervix and then spreads via the pelvic and periaortic lymphatic channels rather than hematogenously. Vascular invasion is usually associated with high-grade, non-estrogen-dependent lesions.

Treatment of endometrial cancer is typically surgical with removal of the uterus, Fallopian tubes and ovaries. Patients with deep myometrial invasion or disease outside of the uterus may be treated postoperatively with radiation, chemotherapy or progestins. Analysis of endometrioid adenocarcinoma specimens for estrogen and progesterone receptor status has recently been introduced into treatment research protocols. There is a good correlation between tumor differentiation and receptor content; greater numbers of both estrogen and progesterone receptors are found in well differentiated lesions than in poorly differentiated lesions. Receptor content appears predictive of response to progestin therapy.

The survival rate for endometrial cancer is relatively good with about a 70% overall survival at 5 and 10 years. Stage I disease, in which the tumor has not invaded through more than half the myometrial thickness, has a 5-year survival rate of over 90%. Because of its high prevalence, endometrial cancer can be considered a neoplasia of high morbidity and relatively low mortality in today's medical environment.

Epidemiology of endometrial cancer

Endometrial cancer is largely a disease of the menopause. About 80% of cases diagnosed are in women between the ages of 50 and 75 years with the peak incidence between 55 and 70 years of age. A 50-year-old American woman has a 2–3% probability of developing endometrial cancer in her remaining lifetime. This number is almost double that observed for carcinoma of the cervix and ovary. The incidence of endometrial cancer is increasing in the United States probably as the result of increasing longevity of the population, earlier and more accurate diagnosis and the increased use of estrogen replacement therapy by menopausal women over the last two decades. The incidence also varies dramatically from country to country, as may be seen in the table below. This geographical incidence follows that of breast and ovarian cancer, with the highest rates in industrialized countries, and is exactly the opposite of patterns observed for cervical cancer.

An association between estrogen exposure and endometrial cancer has been apparent for over 50 years. Many of the risk factors listed in the table on the next page are thought to increase the risk because of their association with high estrogen levels, typically unopposed by progesterone. The single most important and best defined risk factor for adenocarcinoma of the uterus is obesity. Obesity is associated with increased aromatization of adrenal androgens to estrogens by the aromatase activity of adipose tissue, which leads to an increase in circulating estrogens. Obese women also have a lower concentration of sex steroid-binding globulin that increases the bioavailability of the estrogen.

Close links exist between risk of endometrial cancer, a high fat diet and gross national product. This finding suggests that the level of industrial development possibly affects the incidence of endometrial carcinoma by influencing food consumption. A high fat diet is also

Incidence of endometrial cancer in different countries for women selected by age.

Country	Incidence per 100 000
USA (Almeda, CA; white population)	45.8
Germany (Saarland)	33.8
New Zealand (Maori)	28.8
Switzerland (Geneva)	23.6
Canada (Alberta)	21.1
USA (Almeda, CA; black population)	19.3
Malta	17.8
Sweden	16.8
Israel	15.0
Finland	13.4
Poland (Warsaw)	13.2
Romania (Timis)	12.4
United Kingdom (Liverpool)	12.0
Puerto Rico	8.4
Columbia (Cali)	7.0
Singapore (Cinesi)	6.8
Spain (Saaragozza)	5.8
Brazil (Recife)	3.0
India (Bombay)	1.8
Japan (Miyagi)	1.7

Risk factors for endometrial cancer.

Increased risk
Obesity
Diabetes
High fat diet
High socioeconomic status
Urban residence
Positive family history
Polycystic ovary syndrome
Unopposed estrogen replacement therapy in menopause
Tamoxifen use
Estrogen-secreting tumors

Decreased risk
Delayed menarche
Combination oral contraceptive use
Childbearing

associated with obesity and type II diabetes mellitus. Amount and type of dietary fat influences estrogen metabolism as diets rich in beef or fats increase estrogen reabsorption from the bowel.

White women are three times more likely to be diagnosed with endometrial cancer than black women. Again, this is exactly the opposite of what is seen with cancer of the cervix.

Steroid hormones and endometrial cancer

As noted above, the epidemiologic data on endometrial cancer reveal a striking association between estrogen exposure and risk. Interestingly, a direct causal link can only be inferred and has not yet been directly proven. The basis for considering estrogen as an etiologic factor comes from three sources: (i) the biologic activity of estrogen and progesterone on the endometrium; (ii) animal and human data on the effects of diethylstilbestrol (DES) on carcinogenesis; and (iii) the association of endometrial cancer with endometrial hyperplasia and the association of hyperplasia with prolonged and unopposed estrogen exposure.

The strongest attestation to the high sensitivity of the endometrium to ovarian steroid hormones is the dramatic changes that it undergoes in each menstrual cycle (Chapters 9 and 13). The endometrium basically changes its morphology on a day-to-day basis. In the follicular phase of the cycle, estrogens stimulate proliferation of both the epithelium covering the endometrial glands and the underlying stroma. Estrogen induces both its own and the progesterone receptor during this time. Progesterone secreted after ovulation promptly arrests the proliferative activity in the glands and converts the epithelium to a secretory state. The stroma responds to progesterone with angiogenesis and maturation in anticipation of implantation should a pregnancy occur. It is believed that the potent mitogenic effect of estrogen on the epithelium of the endometrial glands accelerates the spontaneous mutation rate of predisposing oncogenes and/or tumor suppressor genes, leading to neoplastic transformation.

In addition to the known mitogenic effects of estrogen on the epithelium of the endometrium, other biologic evidence demonstrating the carcinogenic potential of estrogens in the reproductive tract comes from animal and human data gathered after developmental exposure to

diethylstilbestrol (DES). DES is a non-steroidal estrogen agonist that was among the first synthetic estrogens developed. It was administered to two million women between 1940 and 1970 as treatment for threatened miscarriage. In mice, neonatal exposure to DES produces endometrial cancer in 95% by 18 months of age. In women, prenatal DES exposure lead to structural abnormalities of the reproductive tract (Chapter 25) and to clear cell carcinoma of the vagina and cervix. The carcinogenic action of the DES appears to be mediated in part through activation of the estrogen receptor. Whether prenatal DES exposure will cause endometrial cancer in humans is not yet known because this cohort of women is just entering menopause. The molecular genetic mechanism by which DES and naturally occurring estrogens lead to clear cell carcinoma and type I endometrial cancer, respectively, may be similar. Genetic instability of microsatellite sequences has been demonstrated in both these tumors.

Molecular biology of endometrial cancer

K-*ras* oncogene mutations and microsatellite instability are most common in type I, estrogen-related tumors. Mutations of the *PT53* tumor suppressor gene and overexpression of the *ERBB2* oncogene are more frequently observed in the type II, non-estrogen-related tumors.

Endometrial hyperplasia

Endometrial hyperplasia includes a spectrum of changes in the endometrium which range from a slightly disordered pattern which exaggerates the changes seen in the late proliferative stage of the menstrual cycle to irregular, hyperchromatic lesions that are difficult to distinguish from endometrioid adenocarcinoma. Nonetheless, non-invasive endometrial hyperplasia can be divided into two basic types—hyperplasia and atypical hyperplasia. The atypia consists of nuclear enlargement, hyperchromasia or irregularities in nuclear shape. In addition, lesions are described as simple if the glandular architecture is regular, or complex if the glandular architecture is irregular. Of the four types of endometrial hyperplasias, simple, complex, atypical simple and atypical complex, only atypical complex is at significant risk for progression to invasive carcinoma. About 20% of women with complex atypical hyperplasia will develop endometrial adenocarcinoma compared to 1–2% of those with the other three lesions. The progression from hyperplasia is slow and may take 5 or more years.

Endometrial hyperplasia has the same epidemiologic risk factors as endometrial cancer. Among patients with atypical endometrial hyperplasia, postmenopausal status is associated with the highest risk of progression to adenocarcinoma (33% over 10 years). Endometrial cancer is rare during childbearing years and is usually associated with the polycystic ovary syndrome and chronic anovulation (Chapter 28.2). Estrogen-producing tumors such as the granulosa/theca cell tumors (Chapter 39) are also associated with endometrial hyperplasia and adenocarcinoma in premenopausal women.

Treatment of endometrial hyperplasia with low malignant potential is progestin therapy to stop the proliferation and convert the endometrium to a secretory state. Medroxyprogesterone is usually given either for 10 days per month or continuously. Atypical endometrial hyperplasia is treated with hysterectomy unless there is a contraindication to the procedure.

41 Cervical neoplasia

Overview

Invasive squamous cell carcinoma accounts for 80% of cervical malignancies. If one includes preinvasive lesions, it is the most common genital tract neoplasm. Unlike the remainder of the reproductive tract cancers, which are more prevalent in industrialized countries, cervical cancer is the number one cancer killer among women in the third world. Its epidemiology suggests that it is a sexually transmitted disease. Squamous cancer of the cervix is unique in that it is a preventable disease with proper screening and treatment.

Like prostatic cancer in men (Chapter 38), cervical cancer typically arises from a precursor lesion, cervical intraepithelial neoplasia (CIN). CIN is asymptomatic and appears to precede invasive carcinoma of the cervix by 5–15 years. Almost all cervical cancer arises in the transformation zone (squamocolumnar junction) where the columnar, glandular epithelium of the endocervix meets the squamous epithelium of the ectocervix. The squamocolumnar junction occupies a different position in young postpubertal girls than it does in postmenopausal women (see figure below), making the early diagnosis of cervical neoplasia more difficult in older women in whom the transformation zone may be high in the endocervical canal.

There are three general types of overt cervical cancers. The most common is the large friable exophytic lesion that extends into the vagina and bleeds profusely when touched. Some tumors infiltrate the cervical stroma without outward signs of growth and create 'barrel-shaped' lesions. Barrel-shaped lesions can first present with urinary or bowel symptoms from their local spread. The last category is an ulcerative tumor that replaces the cervix and upper vagina with a large purulent crater.

Cervical carcinomas can spread in any one of four ways: (i) into the vaginal mucosa; (ii) into the myometrium of the lower uterine segment; (iii) into the paracervical lymphatics and from there to the obturator, hypogastric and external iliac lymph nodes; and (iv) directly into adjacent structures such as the bladder, rectum or parametrial tissues extending laterally to the pelvic sidewall. Lymphatic invasion may occur even when the tumor is still small. Hematogenous spread and distant metastases are a very late manifestation of the disease.

Treatment of cervical cancer is surgical for early stage lesions. A combination of radiation and chemotherapy is used for advanced disease and in poor surgical candidates.

Epidemiology of cervical cancer

The association of sexual activity with cervical cancer was first identified over 150 years ago when it was noted that the disease was rare in nuns and frequent in prostitutes. Subsequent epidemiologic data have identified onset of sexual activity in adolescence and multiple sexual partners as high-risk characteristics for cervical cancer. Its incidence is higher in low-income women but this effect is not independent of early sexual activity and many partners. Smoking is an independent risk factor. Characteristics of a 'high-risk' male partner have been identified; men whose previous partner developed cervical cancer or who themselves develop penile cancer put their sexual partner at increased risk.

The epidemiologic data suggesting that cervical cancer behaves like a sexually transmitted disease provoked studies into potential causative agents. Virtually everything that can be found in, or put in, the female genital tract has been implicated as the sexually transmitted agent. The most likely candidate for a causative agent is the human papilloma virus (HPV), although more recent epidemiologic data indicate that HPV infection alone is insufficient. While as many as 85% of cervical cancers contain high-risk HPV sequences, the prevalence of HPV infection in control groups without any evidence of cervical neoplasia is much too high for it alone to account for the cancers.

Pathogenesis of squamous cell neoplasia of the cervix

Because the cervix is so physically accessible, the pathogenesis of cervical neoplasia has been extensively studied. It is clearly a disease caused by vulnerable tissue (the transformation zone) that is exposed to at least one carcinogen and to a degree of host compromise.

The squamocolumnar junction is one of six epithelial boundaries present within the lower genital tract. It is discernible from the 24th week of fetal life throughout adulthood. The position of the squamocolumnar junction is affected by both the hormonal and anatomic changes of puberty, pregnancy and menopause. Prior to puberty, the

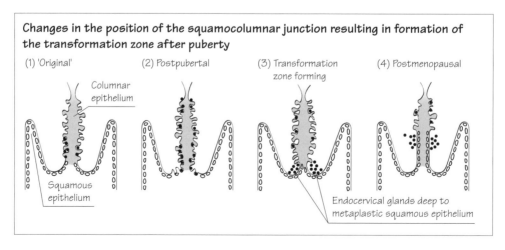

Changes in the position of the squamocolumnar junction resulting in formation of the transformation zone after puberty

(1) 'Original'   (2) Postpubertal   (3) Transformation zone forming   (4) Postmenopausal

Columnar epithelium

Squamous epithelium

Endocervical glands deep to metaplastic squamous epithelium

squamocolumnar junction usually coincides with the position of the external cervical os (Chapter 8). Estrogen-induced changes in the shape and volume of the cervix carry the squamocolumnar junction out onto the anatomic ectocervix, thus exposing the tissues previously found in the lower endocervical canal to the vagina. The exposure of the simple mucin-secreting epithelium to the acidic vaginal environment induces a chemical denaturation of the columnar epithelium exposed at the villus tips. The reparative process, which results from this acidic exposure, eventually produces a mature squamous epithelium. The first sign of the reparative process is the appearance of activated 'reserve cells' beneath the columnar epithelium. The reserve cells gradually become stratified beneath the columnar cells and replace the columnar cells, forming the transformation zone. **After menopause, the squamocolumnar junction retreats high within the endocervical canal.**

Human papilloma virus (HPV) is a DNA virus that causes epithelial lesions in the gastrointestinal tract, skin, cervix and vulva (Chapter 42.3). Its genetic structure is known and two of its nine genes, *E6* and *E7*, appear to have oncogenic potential. It is these sequences that are found in the nuclei of precursor CIN and are integrated into the host chromosomes in invasive cervical cancer. Integration is associated with derepression of genes *E6* and *E7* allowing them to function as oncogenes. The gene products from *E6* and *E7* interact with the tumor suppressor genes, *RB-1* and *TP53*, to disrupt normal growth regulation of host cells. The oncogenic potential of HPV DNA has been demonstrated in the laboratory where it can transform cells *in vitro*.

Of the more than 100 types of HPV identified to date, four are most commonly found in cytologic abnormalities of the cervix including cancers. HPV6 and 11 are associated with low risk for malignancy; by contrast, 85% of cervical cancer contains HPV16 or 18 sequences.

The use of sensitive molecular techniques to ascertain HPV exposure of the genital tract has demonstrated a much higher prevalence of HPV in the general population than was originally reported. Over the last few years, numerous studies worldwide have attempted to reconcile the epidemiology of HPV infection and its oncogenic potential as demonstrated in the laboratory. The current working hypothesis is that the immune response of the host may be key to the development, or lack thereof, of cervical neoplasia from HPV infection. The strongest evidence from this concept is the extremely high incidence of cervical neoplasia seen with cases of blatant immunodeficiency such as is encountered in HIV-infected women and women on immunosuppressive medications following kidney transplants. CIN rates in HIV positive women are 10 times higher than controls and transplant patients have rates approaching 40%. Coinfection with another viral promoter could also explain the failure of epidemiologic data to support the role of HPV alone.

Cervical intraepithelial neoplasia (CIN) is the term used to encompass all epithelial abnormalities of the cervix. It has replaced an older terminology that used the terms 'dysplasia' and 'carcinoma *in situ*' of the cervix. *CIN, although divided into grades, is actually a single neoplastic continuum.* The designations CIN I, II and III are used,

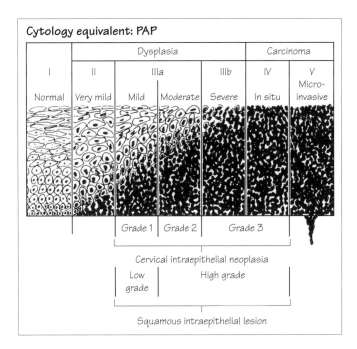

depending on the extent of the cellular aberrations within the epithelium. In CIN I, the lower one-third of the cells lack evidence of cytoplasmic differentiation or maturation. In CIN II, the changes of CIN I occupy two-thirds of the epithelium and in CIN III, the changes are full thickness.

The diagnosis of CIN is made on biopsy specimens taken as part of the evaluation for an abnormal Pap smear screen. Treatment is dependent on the severity of the abnormalities seen in the specimen and other clinical variables.

Pap smear screening for cervical neoplasia

The cervical smear or Pap test (named after Dr George Papanicolaou who developed the test) was designed as a screening test detection of squamous cell CIN. Its success is based on the fact that the nuclear abnormalities of CIN are present in cells that are scraped or exfoliated from the surface of the cervix. Pap smears can also detect cancer, but the detection of a cancer is actually considered a failure of the screening program, which is designed to identify and permit treatment of intraepithelial lesions before they progress to cancer.

Adequate Pap smear screening can reduce a woman's chance of dying from cervical cancer by 90%. Currently it is recommended that all women who are sexually active or have reached the age of 18 have an annual Pap smear screening and pelvic exam. Once three satisfactory normal exams and Pap smears have been obtained, the interval may be increased at the discretion of the woman's physician. Concomitant screening for HPV in the smear may eventually be used to further individualize the appropriate intervals for screening.

42 Sexually transmitted diseases

1 GONORRHEA

Overview

Gonorrhea (GC) is the most frequently reported communicable disease in the United States, but it is an even bigger problem in the developing world where rates 5–50 times higher are reported. The infectious agent responsible for gonorrhea is *Neisseria gonorrhoeae*, a Gram-negative coccus that requires a mucosal surface to gain access to the body. **The major risk of gonorrheal infections is Fallopian tube damage in women, which can result in ectopic (tubal pregnancies) and infertility.**

In men, urethritis is the most common clinical manifestation of gonorrhea. Symptoms include a purulent urethral discharge or dysuria. Between 20% and 30% of heterosexual men with symptomatic gonococcal urethritis are simultaneously infected with *Chlamydia trachomatis*. Local complications of gonorrhea, including urethral stricture, epididymitis and prostatitis, are uncommon in men.

In contrast to gonorrhea in men, gonococcal infection in women is often asymptomatic, but of far greater consequence. A significant number of women diagnosed with gonorrhea are identified in sexually transmitted disease (STD) clinics as the asymptomatic consort of an infected partner. Uncomplicated urogenital gonococcal infection in women may present as dysuria from urethritis, vaginal discharge from cervicitis or purulent drainage from the Skene's or Bartholin's glands at the vaginal introitus. **Pelvic inflammatory disease (PID)** is a term used to describe infection of the upper genital tract and includes endometritis, salpingitis and peritonitis. *N. gonorrhoeae* and *C. trachomatis* are the two most frequently isolated pathogens from women with positive cultures for PID. Women with gonococcal PID present with lower abdominal pain, abnormal uterine bleeding, dyspareunia (pain on intercourse) and fever. Although mortality from PID is low, morbidity is extremely high as it can result in chronic pelvic pain, infertility and tubal pregnancies. In some areas of Africa, as many as 50% of the women are infertile as a result of tubal occlusion from gonococcal PID.

Other serious clinical manifestations include disseminated gonococcal infection (DGI) and gonococcal ophthalmia neonatorum, a severe form of conjunctivitis in newborns who acquire the infection in the birth canal. Neonatal gonococcal ophthalmia can result in blindness if left untreated. It is a rarity in developed countries because silver nitrate or antibiotic occular prophylaxis is mandated at birth, but remains a significant problem in parts of the underdeveloped world.

Treatment of gonorrhea is with antibiotics. The choice of antibiotic has evolved with time because of the propensity of the organism to develop antibiotic resistance and to be associated with other STDs. Guidelines are frequently updated and include two agents such as a β-lactamase-resistant penicillin or quinolone plus tetracycline. Screening for asymptomatic gonococcal infection is part of the routine gynecological and prenatal care of high-risk women because of the potential for serious complications from the infection.

Epidemiology of gonorrhea

Gonorrhea, like chlamydial infections, is largely a disease of youth. The peak incidence is at ages 18–24 years in both men and women. In addition to age, other risk factors for gonorrhea include low socioeconomic status, urban residence, unmarried status, non-white race, male homosexuality and prostitution.

Biology of *N. gonorrhoeae*

Gonococci enter the body by attaching to mucosal non-ciliated columnar epithelial cells through specialized surface structures on the bacteria known as **pili**. Following attachment by the pili, the gonococci then undergo endocytosis by the cell at which time a lipopolysaccharide (LPS; endotoxin)-mediated event kills nearby cells. Following endocytosis of the bacteria, vacuoles containing viable and replicating gonococci pass through the cell from the mucosal surface to the subepithelial membrane, where they are released into the underlying tissue. The surface damage caused by the gonococcus specifically in the Fallopian tube results in the ability of other pathogens, such as chlamydia, to gain access to the upper reproductive tract and cause multiorganism PID. Movement of the gonococci to subepithelial sites also explains the failure to document its presence in the Fallopian tube of a significant number of cases of cervical culture-positive PID.

Gonococci develop their antibiotic resistance through both plasmid and chromosomal mechanisms. Most plasmid mediated resistance is to penicillin and tetracycline while chromosomally mediated resistance is more general and involves mutations altering cell wall permeability or the affinity of antibiotic binding proteins.

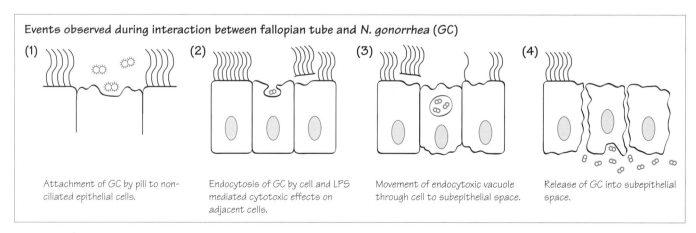

Events observed during interaction between fallopian tube and *N. gonorrhea* (GC)

(1) Attachment of GC by pili to non-ciliated epithelial cells.

(2) Endocytosis of GC by cell and LPS mediated cytotoxic effects on adjacent cells.

(3) Movement of endocytoxic vacuole through cell to subepithelial space.

(4) Release of GC into subepithelial space.

2 CHLAMYDIA

Overview

There are many similarities between the infections caused by *Neisseria gonorrhoeae* and **Chlamydia trachomatis** species. Chlamydiae gain access to the body by invading the same epithelial cells of the endocervix, the urethra, the endometrium, the Fallopian tubes, the rectum and the conjunctivae that are host to the gonococcus. Infections in men are relatively asymptomatic and of low morbidity with both organisms; the major consequence of infection in the male is the risk of transmission to a female consort. In women, gonococcal and chlamydial infections can result in PID, chronic pain, infertility and tubal pregnancy. There is risk to the newborn from a birth canal infected with both gonococci and chlamydiae. The difference is that **chlamydial PID is often asymptomatic. Hence, chlamydial infection is a major public health hazard because of the potential for unrecognized serious damage to the upper reproductive tract of women**.

C. trachomatis is *the* most common STD in the United States. Chlamydiae are unique bacteria that, like viruses, are obligate intracellular parasites and can only be propagated in cell culture. For this reason, knowledge about the extent and nature of chlamydial diseases has lagged behind some of the other STDs.

Chlamydia causes about 50% of the cases of non-gonococcal urethritis in men. In women, chlamydia causes mucopurulent cervicitis and the 'urethral syndrome', in which pain on urination is associated with white blood cells, but no bacteria, in the urine. Unlike gonorrhea, chlamydial infection of the upper genital tract frequently involves the endometrium in the absence of any signs of PID. Chlamydia may cause overt PID, but is also associated with subclinical infection that may first be recognized when the consequent infertility or tubal (ectopic) pregnancy is diagnosed.

Several strains of chlamydia cause a unique disorder known as **lymphogranuloma venereum (LGV)**, a chronic disease that has three stages much like syphilis does. The primary lesion is a small, inconspicuous papule of the genitalia that quickly and quietly disappears. The secondary stage of LGV is characterized by acute lymphadenitis of the inguinal region (bubo formation = inguinal syndrome) and/or acute hemorrhagic proctitis (anogenitorectal syndrome) together with fever and malaise. Most people recover uneventfully from the second stage, but in a few, the chlamydiae persist in the anogenital tissues and incite a chronic inflammatory response which results in genital tract ulcers, fistulae and strictures. LGV is endemic is much of the third world and sporadic in the United States and Europe. In its various stages, LGV is often confused with secondary syphilis, genital herpes and chancroid.

Neonates exposed to chlamydia in the birth canal may develop either conjunctivitis, which can lead to blindness, or a distinctive type of afebrile pneumonia.

Fortunately, chlamydia is sensitive to inexpensive antibiotics such as tetracycline or doxycycline. Unlike gonococci, chlamydiae require prolonged treatment to eradicate the intracellular reservoir of the bacteria. Because of the frequent coexistence of gonorrhea and chlamydial infection, most treatment regimens include one antibiotic to treat the gonococci and another to treat the chlamydia. The quinolones are effective against both, but are currently very expensive compared to the two drug regimens. True antibiotic resistance is rare in chlamydia.

Epidemiology of chlamydial infection

Like gonorrhea, chlamydia infection is a disease of the young. Additional risk factors include low socio-economic status, a high number of sexual partners and oral contraceptive use. Barrier methods of contraception (condom, diaphragm, diaphragm plus spermicide) have a reduced risk; oral contraceptive use may be associated with a higher risk.

Biology of chlamydia

The chlamydiae are structurally complex microorganisms. Like viruses, chlamydiae are obligate intracellular parasites, but are classified as bacteria because they contain both DNA and RNA. They most resemble Gram-negative bacteria in that they possess outer membrane proteins and a lipopolysaccharide (LPS) similar to other Gram-negative bacteria. Chlamydiae are distinguished from all other bacteria by the presence of a unique growth cycle that is characterized by transformation between two distinct forms, the **elementary body** and the **reticulate body**. The elementary body is a highly infectious, rigid

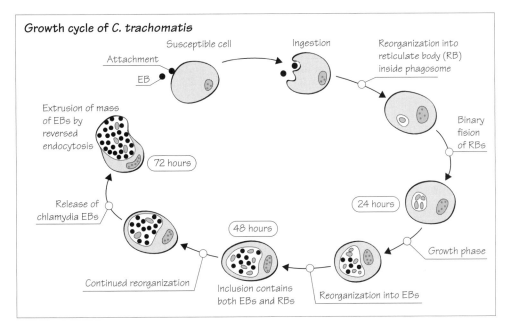

Growth cycle of *C. trachomatis*

Attachment — EB — Susceptible cell — Ingestion — Reorganization into reticulate body (RB) inside phagosome — Binary fision of RBs — 24 hours — Growth phase — Reorganization into EBs — Inclusion contains both EBs and RBs — 48 hours — Continued reorganization — Release of chlamydia EBs — Extrusion of mass of EBs by reversed endocytosis — 72 hours

extracellular growth form that is metabolically inactive. The elementary body attaches to non-ciliated columnar or cuboidal epithelial cells and then induces the host cell to ingest it. The crucial next step in the growth cycle is the failure of the host cell lysosomes to fuse with the elementary body-containing phagosome, thereby permitting the chlamydiae to survive in the cell. Following these two crucial events, the elementary body reorganizes into a larger metabolically active, fragile, non-infectious reticulate body. The reticulate bodies divide repeatedly by binary fission within the phagosome of the host cell, reorganize back into infectious elementary bodies and are released when the host cell dies.

There are 15 different serotypes or serovars of chlamydiae. These serovars are identified as A through K plus Ba and strains L_1, L_2 and L_3. Strains D–K are associated with chlamydial STDs. L_1, L_2 and L_3 cause LGV.

3 GENITAL WARTS

Overview

Genital warts are among the three most commonly diagnosed STDs diagnosed in patients attending STD clinics. They were long considered an inconvenient but benign disease. Since the identification of the infectious agent, the **human papilloma virus (HPV)**, which is responsible for genital warts, and the **association of HPV with genital tract cancers**, the view that genital warts are merely an annoyance has changed.

It is now recognized that there is a broad spectrum of genital HPV infection, which includes (i) latent infection, (ii) subclinical infection, (iii) clinically apparent lesion (condylomata accuminata) and (iv) HPV-associated neoplasia.

Latent infections are identified only by the presence of HPV DNA in tissue samples acquired for epidemiologic study. Subclinical infections are subtle, flat lesions seen with colposcopic examination (microscopic magnification in situ) of acetic acid-treated tissue. Overt genital warts, known also as condyloma acuminata, are flesh-colored, pink or pigmented papules with a frond-like surface. Sessile warts, or flat condyloma-like lesions are less common, accounting for only 20% of visible genital warts. Most genital warts in men are on the penis. In women, they are found most often on the vaginal introitus and labia and less commonly on the vagina or cervix. Except for irritation, most warts are asymptomatic. HPV-associated neoplasias include intraepithelial lesions of the cervix (CIN) and vulva (VIN) and invasive carcinomas in both sites. The role of HPV in cervical neoplasia is reviewed in Chapter 41.

Because most genital warts are sexually transmitted, their presence is a marker for risk for other STDs and patients should be screened for syphilis and gonorrhea. Treatment of genital warts is with either podophyllin, a naturally occurring resin that poisons the mitotic spindle and arrests propagation, or by cryotherapy with liquid nitrogen. Treatment is aimed at removing symptomatic warts because it is not effective in eradicating the virus.

Epidemiology of genital warts

Most genital warts are seen in young people, between the ages of 16 and 25 years. Epidemiologic studies of genital HPV infections are limited because it is now recognized that most infections are subclinical and because there are no sensitive HPV type-specific serologic assays available. Cross-sectional studies on the prevalence of HPV DNA in cer-vical cytologic specimens have shown that 15–25% of women between ages 20 and 25 years are HPV positive with about 5% positive for high-risk subtype 16. By age 35 years, the overall prevalence has decreased to 5% with only 1% positive for subtype HPV16. Penile swabs are HPV positive in about 5% of men.

Most HPV infections are sexually acquired, with about 60% of consorts of patients with genital warts developing the same disease after an average incubation time of 2–3 months. Infectivity appears to decrease over time. It is possible, though rare, to acquire HPV through nonsexual transmission, and neonates can become infected during delivery.

Molecular biology of human papillomaviruses

HPV is a member of the Papovaviridae family of DNA viruses. Other well known Papovaviridae are the polyomaviruses (polio virus and SV40). The virology of HPV has been difficult to study because it is rarely isolated as a free living particle and cannot be propagated in cell culture. Virus-containing material is only available from excised warts. In skin warts, the viral genome is a double-stranded circular DNA molecule. In most HPV-associated lesions, the viral DNA is present as an extrachromosomal episome. In some cancers, the viral DNA is integrated within the host chromosomal DNA.

Of the 70 different HPV genotypes identified, only types 6, 11, 16, 18, 31, 33 and 35 are associated with genital lesions. Types 6 and 11 are most commonly identified in genital warts, and types 16 and 18 with neoplasia (high-risk subtypes). HPV subtypes 1–5 are associated with common and plantar skin warts.

The papillomavirus genome has been extensively analysed. There are nine genes; the functions of eight have been at least partially identified. Genes E1 and E2 are the integration sites into host DNA when it occurs. Genes E1 and E2 function as repressors of genes E6 and E7 in the intact virus; when E1 and E2 integrate, they are disrupted and E6 and E7 are overexpressed. These latter genes are capable of interfering with important tumor suppressor proteins in the host cell, thereby explaining the oncogenic potential of HPV.

Human papillomavirus genes.

E1*	Necessary for viral DNA replication
	May have a role as repressor of immortalization
E2*	Necessary for viral DNA replication along with E1
E3	?
E4	Intracellular protein that interacts with cytokeratin
	? Confers tissue specificity on HPV type
E5	Activates platelet-derived growth factor (PDGF) receptor in host
	Transforms proliferative signal to the cell
E6†	Interacts with p53, a tumor suppressor product monitoring DNA damage
	Transforming signal
E7†	Interacts with Rb-1, the retinoblastoma gene, a tumor suppressor gene that gates the cell cycle
	Strong, transforming signal
L1	Major capsid protein
L2	Minor capsid protein

*Mutations in E1 and/or E2 result in integration of viral DNA into host DNA.
†Disruption of growth regulation necessary to propagate virus.

4 GENITAL HERPES

Overview

Genital herpes is a sexually transmitted disease that doesn't go away. Instead, the responsible agent, **herpes simplex virus (HSV)**, establishes a latent infection in the sacral dorsal root ganglia from which it can be reactivated under a variety of circumstances. The greatest risk of herpetic infection is to the neonate, who acquires it from the genital tract of the mother at delivery, and to immunocompromised patients for whom its disseminated form can be life-threatening. Some studies also link genital HSV infection with risk for cervical cancer, suggesting that it may be a cofactor along with HPV.

There are two distinct serologic types of HSV: HSV-1 and HSV-2. HSV-1 infection is typically asymptomatic, transmitted by primary infection of the respiratory tract, and almost ubiquitous. HSV-1 has been found in the trigeminal ganglion of 80% of cadavers. While HSV-1 reactivation typically causes 'cold sores' or 'fever blisters', primary infection or reinfection with a new strain can cause encephalitis and blinding keratoconjunctivitis.

HSV-2 has a predilection for genital disease, although HSV-1 infections of the genitalia and HSV-2 infections of the oral cavity do occur. HSV-2 is much more likely to become a latent infection of the sacral ganglion and to cause neonatal disease than is HSV-1.

In order to understand the epidemiology and biology of genital HSV infection, it is important to define the three types of HSV infections that can be reported by patients: **primary first episode**, **non-primary first episode** and **recurrent episodes**. First episodes are the first recognized by the patient or health-care provider as genital herpes; recurrences require recognition that the patient has had symptomatic HSV before. Primary first episodes are documented by the absence of HSV antibodies in acute phase serum samples, which prove that there has not been prior HSV infection. Non-primary first episodes are documented by the presence of HSV antibodies at the time of the first recognized outbreak. The severity of clinical manifestations and the incidence of complications at presentation vary according to whether the infection is primary, non-primary or recurrent.

Primary genital HSV disease is the most severe, although it is clear that primary infection can also be totally asymptomatic. Painful lesions on the penis in men and vulva of women, dysuria, urethral or vaginal discharge and painful inguinal adenopathy occur in over 80% of patients. Fever, headache, malaise and myalgias are reported in 40% of men and 70% of women. Urinary retention and proctitis can occur from involvement of the autonomic nerves of the bladder and rectum. Aseptic meningitis occurs in 12–30% of patients. The mean duration of shedding from mucocutaneous lesions in primary genital HSV-2 infections is 2–3 weeks. Non-primary first infections tend to be milder than primary presumably because of acquired humoral and cellular immunity.

Recurrent genital HSV-2 disease typically involves painful recrudescence of the mucocutaneous lesions on the penis or vulva and cervical shedding. Systemic symptoms are absent. The mean duration of symptoms and viral shedding is much shorter with recurrences.

Acyclovir, a purine analog that is a specific substrate for the viral form of the enzyme thymidine kinase, is the drug of choice to treat the symptoms of HSV infection. Treatment with acyclovir will stop viral DNA replication and spread but will not prevent latent infections.

The only prevention for genital HSV infection is abstinence from sexual contact with an infected partner when lesions are visible, although even this is not completely protective as transmission secondary to asymptomatic shedding can occur. Even condoms are not completely protective because the penile shaft may still be exposed to the vulva during intercourse with a condom and because the HSV virus is capable of penetrating latex.

Epidemiology of genital HSV infection

Symptomatic genital HSV infection accounts for 2–4% of visits to STD clinics in the UK and US. It is estimated that about 700 000 new cases of symptomatic first episodes of genital HSV occur in the US each year. Genital HSV infections are reported more commonly among Caucasians than non-Caucasians. Decreasing age at first coitus and increasing number of sexual partners is associated with increasing prevalence of antibody-positive subjects.

The incidence of neonatal herpes is about 1 in every 7500 live births.

Biology of HSV virus

HSV is a member of the herpesvirus class of DNA viruses, which contains two serotypes of HSV (HSV-1 and HSV-2), cytomegalovirus (CMV), varicella zoster (chickenpox, shingles) and Epstein–Barr virus (mononucleosis, chronic fatigue syndrome). Herpesviruses would be better called 'complex' rather than 'simplex' because they have the most complicated structure and replication of all the viruses.

Genital HSV is acquired by sexual contact with contaminated secretions or lesions. Herpesvirus is very susceptible to desiccation and extremes of temperature, making transmission by fomites very rare. Once the virus has gained access to mucosal cells, it destroys the host DNA during productive replication of its own and kills the cell. HSV spreads by contiguity to adjacent cells and tracks toward autonomic nerve endings. Mucosal and skin cells infected with HSV produce serous transudates that result in the classic vesicles seen in the disorder.

After the primary genital mucocutaneous infection, HSV virions travel to the dorsal root ganglia of the sacral plexus (S_2–S_4) via the intra-axonal route where they persist in a non-replicative phase. During reactivation, there is a dramatic increase in DNA synthesis followed by spread of virus back down the sensory neurons to the skin. There are currently two theories of reactivation. In the first, stimuli such as physical injury, hormonal perturbations, immunologic changes or heat, disturb the host ganglion cells to renew DNA synthesis and viral replication. In the second, small amounts of virus are continually produced by the host ganglion cells and travel down the sensory axons to the skin where local conditions determine when a recurrence will occur.

HSV in pregnancy and the neonate

Ninety per cent of women with primary genital HSV-2 infection, 70% of women with primary genital HSV-1 infection and 70% of women with non-primary first episodes of genital HSV-2 infection shed virus from their cervix during the acute infection. This stands in stark contrast to the 12–20% isolation rate for cervical HSV in women with recurrent external genital lesions. Primary genital HSV is associated with a 50% risk of transmission to the neonate; recurrent genital HSV carries less than a 5% risk of vertical transmission. Neonatal herpetic infections are life-threatening and may be prevented with appropriate use of cesarean delivery.

5 SYPHILIS

Know syphilis in all its manifestations and relations, and all other
things clinical will be known to you.

Sir William Osler, 1897

Overview

Syphilis is a systemic disorder with sexual transmission. It is one of
the most fascinating diseases of humans because of its protracted and
variable clinical course. The disease has had great impact on the history
of Western civilization and medical practice. There are two theories as
to the origins of the disease. It is more commonly believed that syphilis
began in the New World, based on the absence of syphilis in skeletal
remains from pre-Columbian Europe and the presence of syphilitic
bones in North and South America. Columbus and many of his sailors
are reported to have been infected during their exploration of the New
World. The late 15th century epidemic of the disease then known as the
'Great Pox' arose from wide spread of the infectious agent during the
ensuing European wars. The alternative explanation, based on descriptions in both the Bible and ancient Chinese writings, is that late cutaneous syphilis was endemic to civilized human populations, but that the
wars and living conditions in Europe perpetuated a more aggressive
form of the disease. An argument against the latter explanation is that
there are several other diseases such as leprosy and tuberculosis that fit
the Old World descriptions.

Natural history of untreated syphilis

Descriptions of the transmission and natural history of untreated
syphilis were provided by several studies early in the 20th century; the
best known are the Oslo study in Norway and the Tuskegee study in the
United States. The latter has been roundly criticized on ethical grounds
because informed consent was not obtained that an effective treatment
was being withheld from the participants.

Syphilis is caused by a spirochete, *Treponema pallidum*, which
enters the body through miniscule breaks in the skin of the external
genitalia that occur during sexual intercourse. Once the spirochete has
entered the body, the untreated disease progresses through **four consecutive stages: primary, secondary, latent and tertiary syphilis**.
Antibiotic treatment at any stage short of tertiary can prevent the late,
life-threatening sequelae of the disease. Syphilis may also be transmitted from a woman to her fetus at any point during pregnancy with
serious consequences.

The primary lesion of syphilis, the **chancre**, develops in venereal
locations close to where *T. pallidum* typically enters the body: the penis
in heterosexual men, the labia or perineum in women and the anus or
rectum in homosexual men. Chancres are painless, small papules that
persist for 1–2 months before healing spontaneously. Swelling of the
inguinal lymph nodes is common. The lesions of primary syphilis may
be confused clinically with herpes simplex, *Streptococcus pyogenes*,
faruncle, chancroid, LGV, granuloma inguinale, histoplasmosis, tuberculosis and squamous cell cancer.

The secondary stage of syphilis is a disseminated form. Blood-borne
spirochetes populate the dermis throughout the body causing a widespread papular rash over the trunk and extremities. Large confluent
papules, known as **condylomata lata**, develop in warm moist areas
such as the vulva, perineum and anus. Because the disease is systemic,
fever, myalgias, lymphadenopathy, sore throat and headache are
common. Secondary syphilis can also be associated with immune complex deposition in the joints, kidneys and eyes, leading to arthritis,
glomerulonephritis, nephrotic syndrome and uveitis. The symptoms of
secondary syphilis can be confused with pityriasis rosea, measles,
infectious mononucleosis, erythema multiforme, leukemia, lymphoma,
ringworm, sarcoidosis and lichen planus.

Untreated secondary syphilis resolves over 4–12 weeks leaving the
patient symptom free. The subsequent months to years until the onset
of symptoms of tertiary syphilis is known as the latent period. The diagnosis of **latent syphilis** can only be made by positive serology (**VDRL**)
in the absence of symptoms or past treatment for syphilis.

Tertiary syphilis usually appears years, often as many as 20–40, after
the disseminated stage. Tertiary syphilis can involve multiple organs,
including the cardiovascular and nervous systems. The most benign
form of late syphilis involves gumma formation in the skin, soft tissues,
bones, cartilage, liver or testes. **Gummas** are macroscopic inflammatory granulomas that develop a central coagulum or 'gummy' necrosis.
Spirochetes often cannot be demonstrated histologically in gummas.
Gummas of the skin are very destructive lesions that leave large ulcers
in their wake. Tertiary syphilis of the aorta results from vasculitis of the
vasa vasorum perfusing the larger vessel. Aortic syphilis leads to aortic
valve insufficiency, left ventricular hypertrophy and congestive heart
failure or aneurysms of the ascending aorta and sudden death. Neurosyphilis can manifest as transverse myelitis, meningitis, dementia,
paresis, optic atrophy and psychosis.

Overall, about one quarter of untreated patients develop recognizable late (tertiary) complications of syphilis, one quarter have asymptomatic lesions demonstrable at autopsy and half have no anatomic
lesions attributable to syphilis present at autopsy. About half of the
patients with symptomatic tertiary syphilis will die as a direct result of
the disease, typically of cardiovascular complications.

Infection of the placenta and fetus will occur in virtually 100% of
women who acquire primary or secondary syphilis in pregnancy due to
the associated spirochetemia. Complications of syphilis in pregnancy include miscarriage, stillbirth, premature delivery and congenital syphilis,
which has a neonatal mortality of 50%. The manifestations of congenital
syphilis are protean.

Signs of congenital syphilis.

Early
Large, thickened placenta
Skin lesions
Enlarged liver and spleen
Fetal hydrops
Disseminated intravascular coagulopathy
Hemolytic anemia
Intrauterine growth restriction
Stillbirth
'Snuffles'
Condyloma lata
Bony abnormalities
Failure to thrive

Late
'Mulberry' molars
'Saddle' nose
'Hutchinson' incisors
'Saber' shins
Hydrocephalus
Mental retardation
Interstitial keratitis

Diagnosis and treatment of syphilis

The diagnosis of primary and secondary syphilis may be made by dark-field identification of spirochetes in scrapings from the skin lesions. Humoral antibodies, detected by non-specific tests such as the Venereal Disease Research Laboratory (VDRL) or rapid plasmin reagent (RPR) assays are present after the primary infection and can be used as a screen for exposure to the organism. Positive VDRL or RPR tests must be followed with a test specific for treponemal surface antigens because of the cross-reactivity of the VDRL and RPR tests with naturally occurring anticardiolipin antibodies.

Treatment of syphilis is with antibiotics, specifically penicillin in all but highly allergic patients. The duration of treatment depends on the stage of the disorder at diagnosis. An unusual reaction called the **Jarisch–Herxheimer reaction** occurs frequently in patients following treatment with antibiotics for primary or secondary syphilis. Symptoms include fever, chills, arthralgias, myalgias, nausea, vomiting and tachycardia. It is a reversible condition caused by sudden death of the spirochetes and either an allergic or endotoxic response to the large antigen load.

Epidemiology of syphilis

Syphilis was a very common disease in many parts of the world until antibiotic therapy became available in the 1940s. Autopsy series indicate that 5–10% of the population of the United States was affected in the first half of the twentieth century. Although antibiotics decreased the prevalence of the disease dramatically after World War II, it began rising again in the 1960s. Currently, the reported incidence is about 15 per 100 000 population with only one-quarter of cases estimated to be actually reported. Women at high risk for contracting syphilis are young, from lower socioeconomic groups and have multiple sexual partners, especially bisexual men. Homosexual men were at extremely high risk for contracting syphilis until the AIDS epidemic increased awareness of the dangers of STDs and changed sexual practices. 10–50 organisms are sufficient to cause infection and about one-third of contacts of an infected person will become infected. The incidence of congenital syphilis parallels that in women and is increasing. Mandatory prenatal screening for syphilis has reduced the incidence of late congenital syphilis; absent or late prenatal care is the biggest risk factor for congenital syphilis.

Biology of *Treponema pallidum*

T. pallidum is a member of the bacterial order *Spirochaetaceae*. *T. pallidum* is closely related to two other treponemas that cause human disease: *T. pertenue*, which causes yaws and *T. carateum*, which causes pinta. Neither electron microscopic examination or DNA analyses can distinguish between these three organisms. It is believed that the different diseases that develop reflect adaptations of the organism and the host to different points of entry into the body.

T. pallidum is a fusilliform organism that cannot survive outside moist areas of the body for more than a few hours. Its microbiology is very poorly understood because the organism cannot be maintained in cell culture. The only animal model for *T. pallidum* infection is the rabbit, which develops the lesions of primary and secondary syphilis, as well as congenital syphilis, after inoculation with the organism.

Most of the manifestations of syphilis are secondary to the inflammatory reaction that the organism causes. Polymorphonuclear cells (PMNs) arriving at the site of the inoculum ingest the spirochetes but do not kill them. Lymphocytes then surround the organism as do macrophages but neither of these cell types kills the treponemes either. Experiments indicate that the infection should be controlled at this point because it is caused by an extremely slow dividing, non-toxin-producing organism surrounded by antitreponemal antibodies and phagocytic cells. Sufficient antitreponemal antibodies are present in the circulation to occasionally cause immune complex glomerulonephritis. It remains both amazing and unknown how *T. pallidum* is able to evade host defenses and establish an infection. The site of primary infection is surrounded by a mucoid material composed of hyaluronic acid and chondroitin sulfate that may alter the host defenses. The best clue available to explain the persistence of disease is the finding that delayed type sensitivity to treponemal antigens is absent in secondary syphilis. New spirochetes inoculated into the system are not infectious while the original infection persists. This is a common mechanism in chronic parasitic diseases called 'premunition'; the host resists reinfection but cannot clear the initial infection.

Subsequent to the establishment of the systemic phase of the infection, the spirochetes are present virtually everywhere in the infected tissues. Inflammation, however, occurs preferentially around small vessels causing intimal hyperplasia and obliterative endarteritis. It is the subsequent focal ischemic necrosis and fibrosis that is responsible for the many late manifestations of the disease.

The inflammatory changes caused by the spirochetes are most striking in congenital syphilis. Congenital syphilis is different from acquired syphilis only in that in acquired syphilis, the lesions are staged in time whereas in neonatal syphilis that follows transplacental fetal infection, essentially all the lesions are part of a single stage of the disease. The placenta is diffusely fibrotic with inflammation and necrosis of the fetal blood vessels in the villi. The resulting vascular insufficiency leads to poor fetal growth (**intrauterine growth restriction**) and **stillbirth**. The fibrosis of the liver and spleen leads to fetal anemia. Subsequent enlargement of these organs, due to compensatory extramedullary hematopoeisis, results in pleural effusions and ascites (**fetal hydrops**). Teeth that form *in utero*, notably the central incisors and the first molars, are infected with spirochetes and the resulting vasculitis affects growth and calcification (**Hutchinson's incisors and mulberry molars**). Ninety-seven per cent of affected infants will have bony lesions caused by gumma formation and destruction of the growth plates. A runny nasal discharge loaded with spirochetes (**snuffles**) may be the only hint of congenital syphilis at birth although some infants also have a skin rash that closely resembles that of secondary syphilis.

The late manifestations of syphilis, both congenital and tertiary, involve vasculitis and parenchymal damage in the central nervous system. In the infant, central nervous system involvement is typically meningovascular and can cause obstructive hydrocephalus. In the adult, the endarteritis of neurosyphilis can cause cerebrovascular accidents, hemiparesis, hemiplegia, aphasia and seizures. Meningovasculitis causes cranial nerve palsies and acute sensorineural deafness. Direct parenchymal invasion of the cerebrum can occur and results in a more generalized symptom complex called **dementia paralytica**, which includes loss of intellectual function, personality changes and psychotic behavior. Periarteritis of nerve ganglia causes **tabes dorsalis** and optic atrophy (**Argyll Robertson pupil**).

Index